THE COMPLETE
ILLUSTRATED
GUIDE TO
ALEXANDER
TECHNIQUE

THE COMPLETE
ILLUSTRATED
GUIDE TO
ALEXANDER
TECHNIQUE

A Practical Program for Health, Poise, and Fitness

GLYNN MACDONALD

mustard

NOTE FROM THE PUBLISHER

*Any information given in this book is not intended
to be taken as a replacement for medical advice.
Any person with a condition requiring medical
attention should consult a qualified practitioner
or therapist.*

Designed and created with
The Bridgewater Book Company Limited

ELEMENT BOOKS LIMITED
Managing Editor: MIRANDA SPICER
Senior Commissioning Editor: CARO NESS
Production Manager: SUSAN SUTTERBY

THE BRIDGEWATER BOOK COMPANY LIMITED
Art Director: PETER BRIDGEWATER
Designers: ALYSON KYLES, KEVIN KNIGHT
Editorial Director: SOPHIE COLLINS
Managing Editor: ANNE TOWNLEY
Editor: KATE QUARRY
Picture research: VANESSA FLETCHER
Three-dimensional models: MARK JAMIESON
Studio photography: GUY RYECART
Illustrators: MICHAEL COURTENAY, IVAN HISSEY,
ANDREW KULMAN

Printed and bound in Italy.

British Library Cataloguing in Publication
data available

Library of Congress Cataloging in Publication
data available

ISBN 1-84164-163-4

Picture Credits

The publishers are grateful to the following for
permission to reproduce copyright material.
AKG: pp 19TR, 110TL, 130BR Allsport: p 147TL
Bridgeman Art Library: pp 34T, 40, 50, 104, 105TL
Cameron Collection: p 30T e.t. archive: pp 20, 67, 70,
117TL, 120BL, 122B, 128, 136B, 178B Image Bank: pp
34BR, 99T, 111TR, 114B, 130CL, 136T, 137, 143, 147,
179, 183 J.P. Kelly: p 47T Rex Features: pp 60, 141 Science
Photo Library: 37BR SIPA Press: p 83 Spectrum: pp 52,
145 ZEFA: pp 46, 49TL, 51, 129, 148, 173, 173, 178T

Acknowledgments

The author wishes to gratefully acknowledge permission to
quote excerpts from the following copyrighted works:
Quotes from F.M. Alexander's book *Articles and Lectures, Man's
Supreme Inheritance* and *The Universal Constant in Living* by
kind permission of Mouritz, ©The Estate of F.M. Alexander
1998. Quotes from F.M. Alexander's *Constructive Conscious
Control of the Individual* and *The Use of the Self* by kind
permission of the publisher Victor Gollancz. Quotes from
Raymond Dart's *Skill and Poise* by kind permission of Jean
Fischer, STAT Books Ltd. Quotes from F.P. Jones *Freedom to
Change* by kind permission of Mouritz.
Quotes from the article 'Enhanced Respiratory Muscular
Functioning In Normal Adults After Lessons in Proprioceptive
Musculoskeletal Education Without Exercise', published in *Chest*
(1992) by kind permission of Joshua Siegal. Quotes from *Indirect
Procedures: A Musician's Guide to the Alexander Technique*
(1997) by Pedro Del Alcantara by kind permission of the
publisher, Oxford University Press. Quotes from *A Means of
Understanding Man* by kind permission of the author Walter
Carrington. Quotes from *Direction: A Journal of The Alexander
Technique* (Vol.2, No.3, 1995) by kind permission of the editor,
Jeremy Chance. Quote from *The Resurrection of the Body* (1969)
by Ed Maisel by kind permission of Thames and Hudson Ltd.
Quotes from *The Lost Sixth Sense: A Medical Scientist Looks at
The Alexander Technique* (1990) by kind permission of the
author, Dr. David Garlick. Quotes from *Fundamentals of Riding:
Theory and Practice* (1995) by Charles Harris by kind permission
of the publisher, J.A. Allen and Co. Ltd. Quotes from *The Neck
and Human Balance* (Thesis, 1995) by kind permission of the
author, Mikael Karlberg. Permission to print the poem *There's a
Hole in My Sidewalk*, ©1993 Portia Nelson, by kind permission
of Beyond Words Publishing Inc. Quotes from *Understanding
Balance: The Mechanics of Posture and Locomotion* (1995) by
kind permission of the author, Dr. T.D.M. Roberts. Quotes from
The Endeavour of Jean Fernal (1946) by Sir Charles Sherrington
by kind permission of the publisher, Cambridge University Press.
Quotes from *The Integrative Action of the Nervous System*
(1961) by Sir Charles Sherrington by kind permission of the
publisher, Yale University Press. Permission to quote from
Nikolaas Tinbergen's article 'Ethology and Stress Disease'
published in *Science* (Vol.185, 1974) by kind permission of the
publisher. Photo of the Royal Academy of Music Symphony
Orchestra © Hanya Chlala reproduced by kind permission of the
Royal Academy of Music. Photo of Raymond Dart reproduced by
kind permission of Frances Wheeler. The photograph of Glynn
Macdonald on back flap by kind permission of John Haynes.

Author's Acknowledgments

I wish to thank my fellow Alexander Teachers who contributed
their knowledge: Peri Aston, Malcolm Balk, Jean Clark, Katarina
Diss, Helene Corrie, Pedro De Alcantara, Graham Griffiths,
Hidemi Hatada, Roger Kidd, Felicity Lipman, Ilana Machover,
Gordon McCaffrey, Tessa Marwick, Sue Merry, Tess Miller,
Daniel Pevsner, Joe Searby, Lori Schiff, Judy Stern, Steven Shaw,
Frank Trembath and Miriam Wohl and to the loyal Alexander
Technique students – Eliza Andrews, Penny Cherns, Pri
Elangasinghe, Anne Freeman, Glen Inanga, Vivien, Sophie,
William, and Alexander Green, Margaret Hubicki, Tony Loyd,
Mary Lutyens and Anna Pallant.
Thanks to everyone at Element Books, especially my Editor,
Caro Ness, and to the Design Team at Bridgewater Books,
especially Andrew Kirk and Guy Ryecart. Special thanks
Elizabeth Atkinson, Dorothea Magonet, John Nicholls, Peggy
Williams and Ros Whalley, and I am grateful to Jean Fischer for
his help with chapters 1-4 and 11.
Finally as William Shakespeare said, "Thanks, thanks and ever
thanks" to Walter and Dilys Carrington, and my husband
Robert Macdonald, and children Jessi and Jack.

CONTENTS

Know Thyself

Know then thyself, presume not God to scan;
The proper study of mankind is Man.
Placed on this isthmus of a middle state,
A being darkly wise and rudely great:
With too much knowledge for the Sceptic side,
With too much weakness for the Stoic's pride,
He hangs between; in doubt to act or rest,
In doubt to deem himself a God or Beast,
In doubt his mind or body to prefer;
Born but to die, and reasoning but to err;
Alike in ignorance, his reason such
Whether he thinks too little or too much:
Chaos of thought and passion, all confused;
Still by himself abused, or disabused;
Created half to rise and half to fall,
Great lord of all things, yet a prey to all;
Sole judge of truth, in endless error hurled:
The glory, jest, and riddle of the world!

ALEXANDER POPE (1688–1744)

HOW TO USE THIS BOOK

The Alexander Technique is often characterized as a kind of physical control drill consisting of a series of rules and regulations – sit up straight, do not slouch, do not cross your legs. Nothing could be further from the truth. *The Complete Illustrated Guide to Alexander Technique* brings together the collective experience of practitioners of the Technique from all over the world to give a fascinating and inspiring picture of this educational therapy. It is not a rulebook; rather it is a program for releasing unnecessary tension and accumulated bad postural habits, encouraging your own self-awareness, and giving conscious control back to the full person

This book is divided into five parts. Part One, **Man's Supreme Inheritance**, gives an account of the history and development of the Technique, and the scientific basis for what has been called the "systematized common sense" of F.M. Alexander's original discoveries. There is a section on the evolution of the Technique and the latest research findings.

Part Two, **The Use of the Self**, describes the basic principles of good use, looking at the way unconscious behavior limits our bodies' natural ability to function efficiently. The key concepts of Conscious Inhibition, Conscious Direction, and Primary Control are explained, and there are sections on the anatomy and physiology of the body. This part of the book concludes with a series of clear step-by-step models of efficient use of the body in performing a range of operations.

Part Three, **Constructive Conscious Control**, shows the Alexander Technique in action, drawing on examples from the performing arts, from sport, and from familiar everyday activities in the home and outdoors. Each example is based on a specific case study.

In Part Four, **The Universal Constant in Living**, the numerous medical and therapeutic benefits of the Technique are detailed, with further case studies. The book finishes by showing how bad patterns can be overcome, and responsibility for yourself regained. There is also a listing of further reading and useful addresses.

BIOGRAPHICAL INFORMATION ABOUT ALEXANDER.

DETAILED ARTWORK ILLUSTRATES THE BASIC PRINCIPLES

The first part of the book gives an overview of F.M. Alexander's discoveries and the subsequent evolution of the Technique.

ALEXANDER'S EARLY EXPERIMENTS ILLUSTRATED

QUOTATIONS FROM ALEXANDER'S WORKS AND THOSE OF OTHER PRACTITIONERS.

INTRODUCTORY TEXT PLACES THE EXAMPLE IN CONTEXT

The second part of the book gives a series of examples of efficient and conscious use of the body in performing different actions.

LISTING OF DOS AND DONTS

STEP-BY-STEP SEQUENCES USING CLEAR PHOTOGRAPHS TO DEMONSTRATE GOOD POSTURE

BOXES GIVE IMPORTANT BACKGROUND INFORMATION

In the third part of the book the lessons of the Technique are related to a range of activities in sport, the arts, and daily life. Each section draws on the experience of teachers and practitioners of the Alexander Technique.

CASE STUDIES DRAWN FROM THE EXPERIENCE OF TEACHERS AND PRACTITIONERS

VARIOUS PROBLEMS IDENTIFIED THROUGH PHOTOGRAPHS

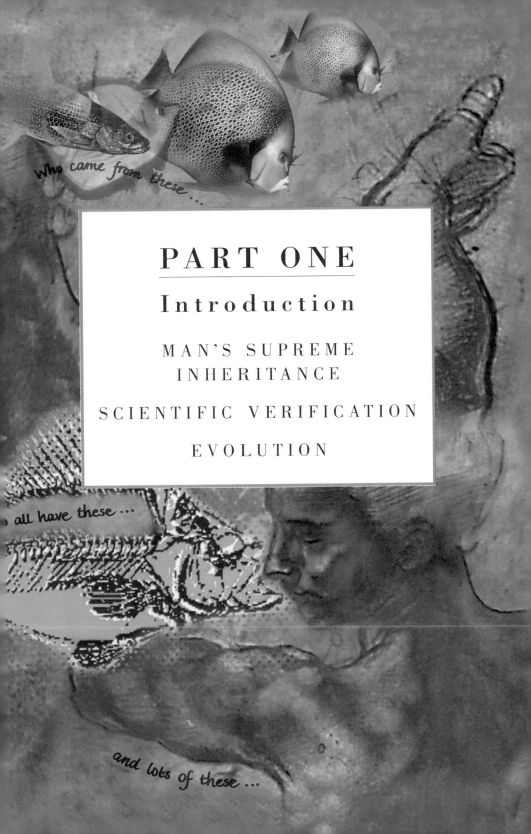

Who came from these …

PART ONE

Introduction

MAN'S SUPREME INHERITANCE

SCIENTIFIC VERIFICATION

EVOLUTION

all have these …

and lots of these …

INTRODUCTION
MAN'S SUPREME INHERITANCE

THE ALEXANDER TECHNIQUE could be described as a method for organizing your sensations of movement, both where you are in space and in time, by becoming more conscious of your internal and external world. You have probably had the experience of feeling run-down, inactive, lethargic, bored, depressed, worthless. Conversely, you have felt as though you were on top of the world – awake and alive,

FREDERICK MATTHIAS
ALEXANDER

everything seeming effortless and wonderful. Conscious guidance and control offer you the possibility to experience a more unified system of efficiency and ease in everyday activities. The Alexander Technique, tested and proved in all walks of life in the last 100 years, recognizes that any action we perform depends for its success on how well the mind and body are functioning in unison.

Our language is full of expressions which reflect the close connection between body and mind, between emotional attitude and physical attitude. We "are on top of things," "feel in good shape," "have a heavy heart," "are scared stiff," "are tied up in knots," "are out of touch," "have a millstone around our neck," "are spineless," "pull ourselves together." These feelings express both our mental and physical state and are easy to discern in our body language. We can recognize someone who is depressed by how they stand, sit, and walk. The joy of a child who is taking its first steps is equally apparent. The joy which a child unconsciously derives from its own "being in action" we too can learn. As we become more "in touch" with ourselves, our knowledge and understanding of ourselves increases. We can become aware of what gets us down and begin to be able to prevent it.

A journey of 1,000 miles starts with the first step.

The Alexander Technique coordinates mind and body in all activities of living. In the process it organizes our sensations of movement, our feelings and emotions, and our experiences of the world around us. It allows us to be conscious of both our "internal" and "external" world. It allows us to be present with all our being. One of the mistakes we make is to assume that the body is disobedient. In fact, our bodies are obedient, but we are frequently unaware of what we are actually asking of them. It is a question not only of being clear about what we want, but of knowing how to ask. To a great extent we have control of our bodies; the Alexander Technique guides control.

When you have conscious control, you can become an originator of life. As you release undue tension, you will release the creativity you possess. You can begin to live in the here and now, conscious of what you are doing, what you are feeling, and with the power to bring about change in yourself and your life. The Technique does not use suggestion, exercises, meditation, or relaxation. John Dewey, the American philosopher of education who advocated "learning through doing," once said of the Technique that it was systematized common sense. When you stop doing the wrong thing and start thinking, the right thing does itself.

Each waking day is a stage dominated for good or ill,
in comedy, farce, or tragedy by a "dramatis persona,"
the self, and so it will be until the curtain drops.
The self is a unity...it regards itself as one, others
treat it as one, the logic of grammar endorses this
by a pronoun in the singular.
All its diversity is merged in oneness.

CHARLES SHERRINGTON

Mind and Body Coordinated

HEAD FORWARD AND UP

BACK LENGTHENED

LUNGS

Poor breathing can be a sign of conflict and tension within ourselves.

Physical poise comes about only when body and mind are harmonized.

The Nature of the mind and soul is bodily; for
when it is seen to push the limbs, raise the body from
sleep, and alter the countenance, and guide and turn
about the whole man and when we see that none of
these effects can take place without touch, nor touch
without body, must we not admit that the mind and
soul are of a bodily nature.

LUCRETIUS: *DE RERUM NATURA*

Modern science separates the living whole into ever-smaller pieces. Experts divide us into the psychological and the physical, the spiritual and the material, the healthy and the unhealthy, and so on. When we seek help, only a part of us is treated. For example, a tennis elbow is treated separately from the entire body poise and the habits of movement that may have caused it in the first place; emotional problems are treated as having a predominantly mental origin.

Tension, general discomfort, poor breathing are all signs of conflict within ourselves, between what we think and what we feel. The more we separate mind and body in everyday activities, the more we lose touch with ourselves: we cease to be able to accurately know what we feel, especially at the very moment it is happening. At worst, our feelings become gross. We only feel the larger events when discomfort and other warning signals have turned into problems, diseases, or "accidents." We can be insensitive and oversensitive; we can block out our feelings as a way of dealing with the stresses of life. A mild or not-so-mild form of sensory deprivation can be the result. We need to respect our senses and appreciate the feedback they give us. Our senses are important because they reflect our state of being; fundamentally they reveal how we are.

FREDERICK M. ALEXANDER
HISTORICAL BACKGROUND AND BIOGRAPHY

FREDERICK MATTHIAS ALEXANDER – the Founder of the Alexander Technique – was born in Australia on January 20, 1869. He came from a family that had succeeded in making a life in a remote outpost on the island of Tasmania, south of the mainland. His background and upbringing made him naturally observant, self-reliant, and disciplined.

In his early youth, one of his chief pleasures was studying the plays of Shakespeare. He became interested in the art of reciting and decided to take it up as a profession, concentrating especially on the great speeches from Shakespeare. In the middle of the last century, electronic amplification did not exist, so performers had to rely solely on the strength of their natural vocal ability. In trying to satisfy the demands that Shakespearean text put upon him as a performer, Alexander began to have trouble with his throat, which affected his voice. He could not control the problem, and at times he lost his voice completely, a medical condition known as aphonia. He consulted doctors and voice trainers, and the medical diagnosis given to him was irritation of the mucous membrane of the throat and nose with inflammation of the vocal cords. The medical advice was that he should rest his voice and speak as little as possible between performances. He followed this advice, but by the time he came to the end of his next recital he could hardly speak, and it

*Speak the speech I pray you,
as I pronounced it to you, trippingly
on the tongue*
WILLIAM SHAKESPEARE: HAMLET

seemed as though his chosen career had come to an end. His doctor suggested that he continue with the resting treatment, but Alexander said he could not go along with this; he had followed advice to rest and his voice had been fine, but after an hour of performing the symptoms had returned. He asked the doctor whether it was not fair to conclude that it was something he was doing in using his voice that was causing the trouble. The doctor agreed, but could not suggest what that something might be. Alexander decided that he must try to find out for himself.

EARLY EXPERIMENTS

Alexander decided to use a mirror to give him feedback and help him see what he was doing while speaking the text. He found that he was continually pulling his head backward when he came to speak. He had not realized that he had this habit. When he began to watch himself more closely, he

The mirror helped Alexander gain the good use necessary for voice production.

*Do not saw the air too much with your hand thus,
but use all gently.*
WILLIAM SHAKESPEARE: HAMLET

discovered that he was lifting his chest, arching his spine, narrowing his lower back, stiffening his legs, and pushing his toes into the floor as well as retracting his head, which was the determining factor in reducing the efficiency of his voice. He said: "I had to admit that I had never thought out how I directed the use of myself, but that I had used myself habitually in the way that felt natural to me."

He began to realize that the mirror was informing him of movements he had not been aware of making, and that he could not trust his feelings. In his book, *The Use of the Self*, he says:

*Discouraged as I was, however, I refused to believe
that problem was hopeless... "Surely," I argued,
"if it is possible for feeling to be untrustworthy as
a means of direction, it should be possible to make
it trustworthy again." The idea of the wonderful
potentialities of man had been a source of
inspiration to me ever since I had come to know
Shakespeare's great word picture: "What a piece
of work is a man! How noble in reason! How
infinite in faculties! In form and moving, how
express and admirable! In action, how like an
angel! In apprehension how like a god! The
beauty of the world! The paragon of animals!"*

LET THE HEAD GO
FORWARD AND UP

HEAD
FORWARD   NECK FREE

Because the majority of the weight of the skull is in front of the spine, the head is naturally inclined to nod forward effortlessly. This allows the neck and spine to lengthen.

LET THE SPINE LENGTHEN

BALANCED HEAD   RETRACTED HEAD

When the head is pulled back and down (retracted), the spine cannot achieve its full length. When the head is in full balance in the same line as the center of gravity, the neck and spine can lengthen.

CONSCIOUS INHIBITION AND CONSCIOUS DIRECTION

Spurred on by the possibility of fulfilling his potential, Alexander continued his experimental work on himself in front of the mirror. Each time he saw he was interfering with his good posture, he would patiently stop. The nature of the control is indirect. If the head is correctly balanced on the body, breathing takes care of itself. In order to achieve this balance, Alexander realized that, first of all, the misuse had to be stopped so he could proceed in a new direction – allowing the neck to be free so that the head could go forward and up, and the back could lengthen and widen. These directions changed the whole use of the body, leading to improved functioning.

These directions are only possible if the inhibitory process is set in place first (*see, Conscious Inhibition page 33*). Inhibition is the key to conscious control of direction. He needed to stop for a second and detach himself from the stiffening and contracting that was occurring inside him. When he calmed down the unnecessary internal activity, then he could stop holding his breath and objectively decide not to react mindlessly. This allows the level of tension that often precedes any action to be reduced. Alexander had discovered that if he could stop the wrong habits, then the right direction could happen.

Gradually he began to develop an understanding of how his head, neck, and back could work

Let the head go forward and up. The gentle hands of the teacher prevent the pupil from pulling her head back and down and restricting her breathing.

Let the breath return freely. The hands of the teacher remind the pupil not to collapse down in front as she breathes out.

Let the back lengthen and widen. The pupil begins to stand in a balanced way, at her full height.

Release me from my bands with the help of your good hands
WILLIAM SHAKESPEARE: THE TEMPEST

Alexander Technique teachers help their pupils to experience Conscious Inhibition and Direction.

harmoniously together and in what ways he was interfering with that optimum functioning. The inflammation of the vocal cords disappeared and his voice became reliable and effective. His general health also improved. By an indirect route Alexander had made a significant scientific discovery. Professor John Dewey said in his Introduction to *The Use of the Self*:

> *I cannot speak with too much admiration of the persistence and thoroughness with which these extremely difficult experiments and observations were carried out. In consequence, Mr. Alexander created what may be truly called a physiology of the living organism.*

The sucking and gasping for air which had so bothered him stopped, and his breathing improved greatly. He then realized that imperfect breathing was not limited to those with vocal problems but applied to most people.

Good posture relieves pressure on the internal organs, allowing them to function properly.

CONSUMPTION

In the 19th century, consumption, also known as respiratory tuberculosis, was the single most common cause of death. Rising living standards and improved hygiene made the incidence of the disease decrease, but at the turn of the century the only treatment available was rest, good diet, and as much fresh air as possible. In 1903, Alexander wrote an article entitled, "The Prevention and Cure of Consumption," in which he described his "art of breathing," listing the following benefits from the practice of his Technique.

Lungs

1. A far greater quantity of air is inspired into and expelled from the lungs.

Oxygenation

2. The oxygenation of the blood is more adequate.

"Vital Capacity"

3. The "vital capacity" is greater.

Thorax

4. The mobility of the thorax is increased daily.

Lung Tissue

5. The lung tissue is nourished in much greater degree.

Digestion

6. The digestive organs are stimulated to an unusual

Respiration

7. The strain in respiration and speaking is removed from the throat.

Breathing

8. Nasal breathing (night and day) is firmly established.

Heart

9. The heart's action is improved daily.

SCIENTIFIC VERIFICATION
OF THE ALEXANDER TECHNIQUE

FROM THE BEGINNING doctors and scientists realized that Alexander had discovered a fundamental principle in human movement and behavior. During Alexander's lifetime several doctors testified to the effects of his technique in journals like *The Lancet*, and, in 1937, 19 doctors urged in a letter in the *British Medical Journal* that the Alexander Technique should be included in medical training (*see page 23*).

One of the principles of the Technique is that use affects functioning; that is, the way we "use" ourselves (move, think, etc.) affects how well we function. A second principle is that the organism functions as a whole. So the execution of a specific movement reflects the overall functioning of the organism. Sir Charles Sherrington confirmed Alexander's treatment of this issue when he wrote in *The Endeavour of Jean Fernel*:

> *In urbanized and industrialized communities, bad habits in our motor acts are especially common. But verbal instruction as to how to correct wrong habits of movement and posture is very difficult. The scantiness of our sensory perception of how we do them makes it so ... Mr. Alexander has done a service to the subject by insistently treating each act as involving the whole integrated individual, the whole psychophysical man. To take a step is an affair, not of this or that limb solely, but of the total neuromuscular activity of the moment – not least of the head and neck.*

Sir Charles Sherrington

Sir Charles Sherrington (1857–1952) was an English physiologist whose researches on reflex action, and especially *The Integrative Action of the Nervous System* (1906) constituted a landmark in modern physiology. He was awarded the Nobel Prize in 1932.

This applies equally to learning: how well we learn depends on well we are. As the great educationalist John Dewey said: "The Alexander Technique bears the same relation to education as education bears to life."

A third principle of the Technique states that the relationship between the head, neck, and back has a paramount influence on the whole organism, its posture and health. Scientific support for this contention came in the 1920s with the publication of Professor Magnus' experiments with animals which suggested that the head–neck–back relationship had a dominating influence on the position and attitude of the rest of the body.

Several eminent scientists have testified to Alexander's scientific method and results. Raymond Dart, the famous anthropologist, wrote in his book *Skill and Poise* that:

> *electronic facilities have confirmed Alexander's insights and authenticated the Technique he discovered in the 1890s of teaching both average and skilled adult individuals to become aware of their wrong body use, how to eliminate handicaps and thus achieve better (i.e. increasingly skilled) use of themselves, both physically and mentally.*

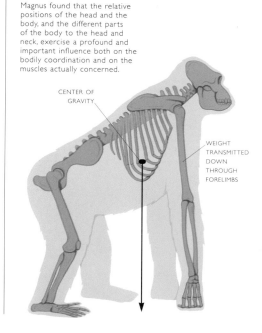

Magnus found that the relative positions of the head and the body, and the different parts of the body to the head and neck, exercise a profound and important influence both on the bodily coordination and on the muscles actually concerned.

CENTER OF GRAVITY

WEIGHT TRANSMITTED DOWN THROUGH FORELIMBS

In his acceptance speech for the Nobel Prize for Medicine in 1973, Professor Nikolaas Tinbergen spoke of the importance of Alexander's work. He noted:

very striking improvements in such diverse things as high blood pressure, breathing, depth of sleep, overall cheerfulness and mental alertness. resilience against outside pressures, and... in such a refined skill as playing a musical instrument.

REPRINTED WITH PERMISSION FROM *SCIENCE* (1974), AMERICAN ASSOCIATION FOR THE ADVANCEMENT OF SCIENCE

Nikolaas Tinbergen

Nikolaas Tinbergen (1907–1988) was one of the founders of modern ethology: the study of animals' behavior in their natural environment, incorporating both evolutionary and social factors.

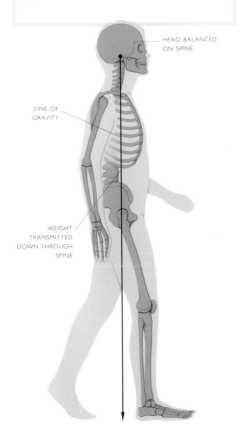

HEAD BALANCED ON SPINE

LINE OF GRAVITY

WEIGHT TRANSMITTED DOWN THROUGH SPINE

Rudolf Magnus

Professor Rudolf Magnus (1873–1927) was a Dutch physiologist whose experiments in the Netherlands found that any interference with the control mechanism concerned with the use of the head and neck in relation to the trunk modified and changed the use of the limbs. Magnus demonstrated that head-neck reflexes were the central mechanism in orienting the animal to its environment.

In addition to personal testimonies, numerous scientific studies have been conducted into the workings and effects of the Technique over the years. Dr. Wilfred Barlow's experiments showed an improvement in posture after lessons in the Technique (postural faults were of course independently assessed). Another experiment conducted by Dr. Barlow in the 1950s showed how the Technique improved the performance of music students at London's Royal College of Music. In the 1960s Professor F. P. Jones in Boston showed how the Technique brought about smoother, more efficient movements by recording movement patterns. He also measured muscle activity (EMG) and demonstrated that

Pedro de Alcantara, the cellist and author of *Indirect Procedures*, shows the benefits to be gained in performance terms from improved posture.

subjects employing the Technique used less muscular effort. This was a confirmation of the feeling of lightness and ease that is a common experience for everybody who practices the Technique.

In the late 1980s Dr. David Garlick's studies at the University of New South Wales showed that when the postural muscles of the back increase in activity to maintain the upright posture, then the trunk muscles are freed, resulting in improvement in respiration. He writes in *The Lost Sixth Sense*:

> *Our studies of subjects, who showed higher levels of electrical activity in their back muscles, also showed... slower and deeper respiratory movement. The interpretation was that, as the back muscles were more active in maintaining the trunk of the upright person, this freed the muscles of respiration – thoracic and abdominal – so that they were able to serve their main function of respiration since they were not required for trunk support.*

He also wrote that the Technique

> *...has relevance for the musculoskeletal system and for ease of posture and movement, preventing problems arising in the body and has important implications for one's emotional state, one's moods.*

In 1992 Dr. John Austin published his study of the Alexander Technique's influence on breathing. He concluded that it demonstrated "a strong association between a course of Alexander Technique instruction and an increase in measures of respiratory muscular strength and endurance." He also identified four possible mechanisms to account for the changes.

1. Increased length of the muscles of the torso.
2. Increased strength and/or endurance of muscles of the abdominal wall.
3. Decreased resting tensions of chest wall muscles.
4. Enhanced coordination of the respiratory muscles.

David Garlick

David Garlick (1933–) is a Medical Scientist heading the Laboratory for Musculoskeletal and Postural Research at the School of Physiology and Pharmacology at the University of New South Wales, Australia.

Austin saw these changes as indirect results of the lengthening in stature and the "subjects developing particular appreciation of head neck elongation and poise."

T.D.M.Roberts

Dr. Tristan Roberts, formerly Reader in Physiology at the University of Glasgow, has a wealth of experience in the mechanisms of Balance, Posture, and Locomotion.

Roberts says in *Reflexes, Habits and Skills*:

> *The correction of some postural habits can significantly improve a person's well-being. For example, many people exert additional effort to supplement the muscular actions called for in maintaining uprightness and in supporting the limbs. As this extra effort frequently involves simultaneous activity in opposing muscle groups, the effect is to stiffen the joints and cause undue fatigue and even pain. To correct such habitual*

Maintaining good posture requires an awareness of our selves.

inappropriate muscular activity, the therapist must somehow induce the patient to become aware of the proprioceptive signals that initiate the unwanted activity. If this awareness can be achieved, the patient is provided with an opportunity of voluntarily refraining from initiating the stiffening actions. His posture thereafter becomes more supple and, consequently, more comfortable to maintain.

A NEW DISCOVERY

Alexander's discovery is comparable to the discoveries made in the Renaissance that caused men to change their ideas of external nature. When you look through a microscope or a telescope for the first time, if you accept the evidence of your senses, you will revise your views of the universe outside yourself. Alexander discovered a way of using his hands to give a person new experiences that force him to revise his ideas both of himself and of the universe. Of course, a person can reject the experience just as the professor of philosophy at Padua rejected Galileo's hypothesis by refusing to look through the telescope. The important thing is that the experience is now available, thanks to Alexander's discovery.

Like the discoveries of the Renaissance, Alexander's ideas can change our view of the world.

Good use of the body prevents overexertion, strain, and fatigue.

Movement becomes energized and poised without unnecessary stiffening.

EVOLUTION

When he speaks
The air, a chartered libertine, is still
And the mute wonder lurketh in men's ears
To steal his sweet and honeyed sentences ...
  WILLIAM SHAKESPEARE: *HENRY V*

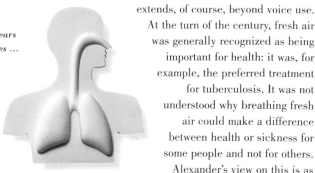

ALEXANDER SOON BECAME known
as the "breathing man"
because of his ability
to breathe effortlessly and
noiselessly when acting or
reciting. The importance
of the freedom of breathing

extends, of course, beyond voice use.
At the turn of the century, fresh air
was generally recognized as being
important for health: it was, for
example, the preferred treatment
for tuberculosis. It was not
understood why breathing fresh
air could make a difference
between health or sickness for
some people and not for others.
Alexander's view on this is as
simple as it is obvious.

What really makes a difference is the amount of oxygen that is pumped around by the blood. Breathing is the process not only of bringing air into the lungs, but also of transporting the oxygen around so it can reach the cells that need it. The Alexander Technique not only brings about deeper and calmer breathing, but because all the muscles are releasing and expanding, it allows the blood – and thereby oxygen – to flow uninterrupted. In this way, breathing becomes easy and the efficient blood-flow ensures oxygen is pumped around everywhere.

In an article for the Sydney *Daily Telegraph* in 1903, Alexander pointed out that the decline of the "breathing power of mankind ... is unquestionably one of the most striking features of our modern civilization." He criticized the then fashion of "deep breathing" as a mechanical, thoughtless exercise. The idea of taking a deep breath is simply counterproductive. Similarly, chest exercises do not increase the amount of air capacity; they simply lift the chest, build muscles on the outside of the ribs, and make the chest look bigger. For an expansion and enlargement of the lungs to happen, the whole body needs to release and expand. In daily life, i.e. in activity, this can only happen when the whole muscular system is coordinated.

We say that a person is a bad breather or that he breathes imperfectly, but this so-called bad breathing is only a symptom and not a primary cause of his malcondition, for the standard of breathing depends upon the standard of general coordinated use of the psychophysical mechanism. What we ought to say, therefore, in such a case is not that a person breathes badly but that he is badly coordinated.

Henry Irving (1800–1900), a great actor who claimed he did not have a single natural attribute for becoming an actor.

When doctors realized that Alexander had discovered something new and remarkable, he was persuaded to introduce his method in London, where he moved in 1904. He soon established a thriving practice, initially teaching members of the theatrical profession, but also people who had been recommended by their doctors to see him. In the early evening he would travel between West End theaters, helping actors to prepare for their performances (among them Henry Irving, Herbert Beerbohm Tree, and Lily Brayton).

In 1909 the Alexander Technique was proposed as a physical education system for Australian schools. Commissioned by the Australian Board of Education, Dr. A. Leeper examined methods of physical education

Walter Carrington

Walter Carrington (1915–) is joint director with Dilys Carrington of the Constructive Teaching Centre, London. He found that it is in the sphere of education that the Alexander Technique will find its most important application. People taught on this basis will be able to answer the question "How do I best set about doing what I want to do?" Their knowledge of the Technique will give them such a practical working knowledge of the human organism that they will not be misled into believing that life is normally conducted along rational lines, or that it is only necessary to think rationally in order to act rationally. They will have had sufficient experience in the difficulties of controlling their own reactions to know that the process of conscious reasoning is not easily cultivated and also that it can only be cultivated by means that take into account the functioning of the organism as a whole.

in England and concluded in his report that he would "without hesitation" give "the first place to the system associated with the name of Mr. F. Matthias Alexander." He wrote:

The results are most striking. It's no exaggeration to say that most of the leaders of the dramatic profession in London (and what better judges could possibly be found?) are enthusiastic believers in the efficacy of his system, and many of them have placed themselves under him for tuition… I also wrote to several specialists in London, who have been sending patients to Mr. Alexander for the cure of defects of speech, throaty vocalization, and chest weakness. They one and all speak of his results as entirely satisfactory.

Despite this warm recommendation Dr. Leeper's advice was ignored by the Australian School Board. However, Alexander received much encouragement from many other people. For example, his holistic view of health was publicly supported by Dr. J. E. R. McDonagh in his three-volume work *The Nature of Disease* (1931–36). McDonagh agreed with Alexander's observation that the wrong use of the body played an important role in the nature of disease and suggested that Alexander's work could be described as the first clinical physiology for the human being. Alexander was further encouraged with the success of his first book, *Man's Supreme Inheritance*, in 1910.

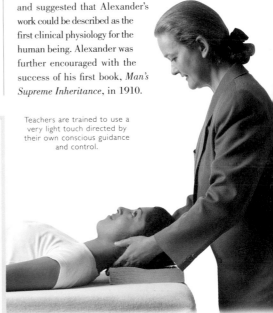

Teachers are trained to use a very light touch directed by their own conscious guidance and control.

Training and Qualifications

There are over 2,000 Alexander Technique teachers throughout the world, with 1,000 students undergoing a three-year Training Course Program. This thorough training leads to qualification as a teacher of the Alexander Technique and approved membership of S.T.A.T., the Society of Teachers of the Alexander Technique.

ALEXANDER'S WRITINGS

1910 MAN'S SUPREME INHERITANCE

In 1910 Alexander published *Man's Supreme Inheritance* in which he proposed an evolutionary explanation for the general deterioration in health and well-being of modern man. The course of evolution had allowed adaptation to be a gradual one. Man's present state reflected his inability to adapt himself to the rapidly changing circumstances of civilized life. Reliance on subconscious guidance of the mental and bodily processes was no longer successful. Our "supreme inheritance" was the possibility of passing from subconscious to conscious control of ourselves. He argued against the unconscious pursuit of exercise, relaxation, and deep breathing methods as remedies because they did not deal with the underlying cause of misuse, which was unreliable sensory appreciation.

Alexander advocated the study of conscious control and its universal application to the eradication of habits of misuse. It involved:

a) an ability consciously to inhibit habitual interference with the upright posture

b) an ability freely to control the motivating factors responsible for misusing the body, as well as an ability to consciously direct the body into an efficient posture and working state

c) an ability to maintain improved functioning in all activities, especially when facing unfamiliar circumstances

Before conscious control could become a reality, it was necessary to recognize the conflict that existed between impulsive reactions and reasoned conceptions.

Because of the unity of mind and body, a habit could never be thought of as simply mental or physical, but recognized as a unified response of the whole self. A habit involved a deterioration of the muscular sense that makes it difficult to distinguish between appropriate and inappropriate effort, a need for the habit, and mental resistance or laziness of some kind.

Changing habits required a recognition of true body poise, together with an understanding of the inhibitory and volitional powers of the mind.

1924 CONSTRUCTIVE CONSCIOUS CONTROL

In 1924 Alexander published *Constructive Conscious Control of the Individual*. In this second book, he discussed sensory appreciation in its relation to evolutionary development, and human beings' needs and happiness. Approaches to learning and learning to do were also incorporated.

Our ancestors had displayed good body use, which was controlled by instinct. However, these instincts did not equip them for the rapid advances and changing circumstances of modern civilized life. He argued that, on the whole, we lacked the grace and poise of our ancestors, and often displayed poor body use and an inability to efficiently change our posture. Restoration of sensory appreciation to a reliable standard was essential.

Alexander introduced the term "end-gaining." It was used to describe directly proceeding to gain a desired end which resulted in an unsatisfactory use of ourselves. Alexander suggested adopting the principle that he termed "the means whereby." This involved a willingness to pay attention to the process with which an end is achieved, resulting in a more satisfactory use of ourselves.

He argued that our conception of an idea or an instruction depends on our standard of sensory appreciation. Most teaching overlooked this fact as it was based on the incorrect assumption that having asked someone to do something, they will be able to do it. He exposed the fallacy of correcting a defect when sensory appreciation was unreliable and advised the re-education of the whole person. A recognition of this unreliable sensory appreciation was the first step to correcting a defect instead of simply doing something else which might have been equally wrong.

During the process of learning the Alexander Technique, pupils began to stop end-gaining and trying to be right. This principle of prevention was central to the understanding and practice of the work. In a discussion on the problem of concentration, he argued that the inability to attend to two things at once is an indication of poor sensory appreciation resulting in misdirected effort.

1931 THE USE OF THE SELF

In 1931 he published *The Use of the Self* in which he described in detail the process of developing his technique. He covered the time from when he discovered that his loss of voice was caused by an instinctive misuse of his body to when he overcame his wrong habitual use.

Along the way he made some important observations concerning human behavior. They included the influence of use upon functioning, the primary control, the fact that instinctive misdirection was associated with the untrustworthiness of feeling and an instinctive response to stimuli. He reasoned that feeling could be made trustworthy again. The application of his technique was illustrated in two case histories: that of a stammerer and a golfer. He explained the extent to which we are dominated by habit, and the importance of learning to prevent old habitual responses in order for new responses to happen.

In the Chapter "Use and Functioning in Relation to Reaction," Alexander discussed how our reflex functioning and our reactions to stimuli were conditioned by the use of the whole self. As a result of an increasingly untrustworthy sensory appreciation, the direction of the body, which is monitored and organized by instinct, has become more and more a misdirection, resulting in symptoms of mental disorder, disease, and poor reflex functioning. By teaching the technique of conscious redirection of the stature, general functioning could be indirectly improved.

He explained that his technique did not involve dealing with specific symptoms directly, but established a more satisfactory general direction of use which was the basis for improved psychophysical functioning. One critic, trying to explain the vitality of these books over so long a time said, *"These are books not for a day or a year, but for all time."*

1941 THE UNIVERSAL CONSTANT IN LIVING

In 1941 he published *The Universal Constant in Living*, where he discussed the manner of use as exerting a "constant" influence over general functioning and reaction. The fact that muscles are constantly being used affects our health. He argued that we can coordinate and control that use to our best advantage.

In the Chapter "The Constant Influence of Manner of Use in Relation to Diagnosis and Disease," Alexander discussed medical case histories he had experienced. A letter, quoted in the *B.M.A. Journal* of 1937 and signed by 19 eminent doctors of the time, says:

We are convinced that Alexander is justified in contending that an unsatisfactory manner of use, by interfering with general functioning, constitutes a predisposing cause of disorder and disease, and that diagnosis of a patient's troubles must remain incomplete unless the medical man, when making the diagnosis, takes into consideration the influence of use upon functioning.

In the Chapter "A Review of the Report of the Physical Education Committee of the British Medical Association," he pointed out the fallacies and limitations of physical exercise. Alexander criticized the B.M.A. report as taking the reliability of individual sensory appreciation for granted. He stated that the performance of exercises, while still under the influence of unreliable sensory appreciation, using the very sensory processes that need correction, could not be beneficial and tended to aggravate the problem.

Alexander encouraged his pupils to inhibit their response to any stimulus. Simple, everyday activities, such as sitting down in a chair or getting up from a chair, allowed pupils to have a new sensory experience of a more upright stature with the accompanying sense of increased freedom in movement.

Alexander used the example of a golfer to show how habitual body postures can interfere with performance.

THE SOCIETY

A FEW YEARS BEFORE F. M. Alexander's death, discussions began about the formation of a professional society to supervise standards of teaching and teacher training, and in 1958 the Society of Teachers of the Alexander Technique (S.T.A.T.) was formed in Britain with the following aims:

1. To maintain and improve professional standards.
2. To make the Technique more widely known.
3. To facilitate contact between members.
4. To encourage research.
5. To prevent abuse and exploitation by untrained people.

At that time, in 1958, three Alexander teacher training courses had been running in Britain. By 1997 there were 14 approved by S.T.A.T. in the U.K., and courses in at least nine other countries approved either by S.T.A.T. or by similar professional societies set up more recently in those countries. The Society assesses the suitability of those who wish to run teacher training courses and lays down minimum requirements in terms of length of training, structure of training, and core curriculum. There is also a system of visits by external moderators to try to maintain equivalence of qualification standards among courses. Because the nature of the work is so individual, courses are small, ranging from 5 to 40 trainees, and a teacher–student ratio of about 1:5 is recommended. Classes usually take place for 3–4 hours a day, four or, more commonly, five days a week, still following the basic pattern established by Alexander himself, as that level of consistency and continuity has been found to be most beneficial.

John Nicholls, Director of the Brighton Alexander Training Center, instructs his student in the refined use of her hands and directed use of herself.

TRAINING COURSES
JOHN NICHOLLS

Make it your ambition to lead a quiet life, to mind your own business, and to work with your hands.

I THESSALONIANS 4: 11

AN OLD JOKE AMONG students on Alexander teacher training courses goes something like this. Student arrives home looking weary after morning on the training course. Partner asks sympathetically: "You look worn out. What did you do in class today?" Student replies: "Oh, I lay on the floor for a while, then I went in and out of a chair a few times, walked a few steps, lay down again, sat with my hands on the back of another chair, and then put my hands on someone else while they stood up and sat down. I'm absolutely exhausted!"

Indeed, to anyone unfamiliar with the process visiting an Alexander teacher training class, that is rather how it might look: a group of people repeatedly performing mundane, simple activities with great care and attention. Not exactly a hard day on the factory floor! Yet the tiredness is real, especially during the first year of the training, as these simple procedures put demands on muscles to work in new ways, and the clarity of attention required is almost like building up new "mental" muscle.

Alexander's first attempts at training others to teach his work were of an informal apprenticeship nature. His brother A. R. and his sister Amy had assisted him in Melbourne, and in London he took on Ethel Webb and Irene Tasker as assistants in a similar fashion. However, in 1931 a more organized training program began. From the beginning it was a three-year program, with students meeting for several hours, five days a week, during the typical British educational term-times. The emphasis was largely on students working to develop their own use of the Technique to a very high level, as Alexander firmly believed from his own experience of teaching that you must practice what you preach.

In the work of kinesthetic (or sensory) re-education, the good use of the teacher is the paramount factor determining whether his hands succeed in conveying to the pupil the sensory experience of the coordination required, and only personal experience can enable a teacher to give the clear verbal explanations that are also necessary.

The attention required to re-educate the body develops a kind of "mental muscle."

This basic training format continued until Alexander's death in 1955, when the original course was carried on by Walter Carrington. In subsequent years Walter and his wife Dilys Carrington have maintained this direct link with Alexander, and added extra structural elements to the training, such as regular study of Alexander's books and other relevant literature, study of anatomy and physiology, and a more organized approach to the development of the manual skills of Alexander teaching. The majority of the training courses operating today proceed along these lines.

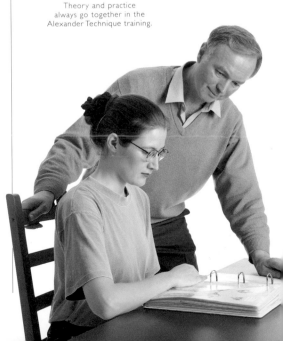

Theory and practice always go together in the Alexander Technique training.

Learning for Life

When someone is having individual lessons in the Alexander Technique, a process of change and improvement takes place by frequent repetition of simple activities under the guidance of the teacher. Emphasis is on the quality of attention to the pupil's use of the Technique as the activity is performed, so the ends to be gained may seem relatively easy, but the quality of performance is all-important, rather than success. An analogous process takes place in the training of Alexander teachers. The actual maneuvers a teacher performs with hands on a pupil really look quite simple: moving someone in and out of a chair; gently holding and guiding their head, neck, torso, and limbs in sitting, standing, and while the pupil lies on a firm couch. Can this really take three years to learn, especially when compared to the apparently complex manual skills of, say, osteopathy or chiropractic? But as with the individual lesson process, the secret lies in the quality of performance: learning to do simple things with a very high degree of coordinated use; the teacher's whole body expressing the light, lively, integrated, elastic muscle tone he or she is aiming to convey to the pupil. This is not just a matter of being a good visual role model. We have found from many years' experience that the "tone" of the experience conveyed by the teacher's hands is a reflection of the tone of the teacher's entire body. The external simplicity hides a skill that will go on being refined throughout the teacher's working life.

A teacher therefore has to learn to achieve this coordinated expansion with hands on a pupil, and to maintain it while doing any further necessary muscular work, moving a pupil's head, arm, or leg, for example. Thus any muscular activity required on the part of the teacher is spread throughout his whole body, not producing a buildup of shortened, tense muscle in any one part. This way of working constantly conveys a releasing, integrating, expansive stimulus to the pupil, both at rest and in movement.

Even while they teach, men learn.

SENECA: *EPISTULAE MORALES*

The experienced hands of the teacher allow the appropriate release to happen.

Use of Hands

Alexander Technique teachers give precise verbal instructions reinforced by use of their hands. In most forms of what might be termed "manual therapy," for example, physiotherapy or osteopathy, there are two distinct modes of using the hands. They are used to feel, to palpate and discover what the problems are in the patient; then they are used to intervene, to perform some type of manipulative maneuver to correct the perceived problem. A distinct feature of good Alexander teaching is that these two modes are unified: that use of the teacher's whole self that makes for greatest sensitivity in the hands to feel what is happening in the pupil is at the same time the key aspect of conveying to the pupil the possibility of change to a better manner of use.

One of Alexander's most useful discoveries was the practical procedure known as "Hands on the back of the chair." It provides a paradigm for all use of the hands in activity, ensuring that the use of the hands is coordinated with the primary needs of the trunk for upright support and freedom to breathe. Alexander himself is often quoted by teachers who trained with him as saying this procedure contained all the experiences one needed to use the hands as a teacher of the Technique. The hands on the back of the chair procedure therefore provides the background to all the learning required to use one's hands on others in an Alexander teaching program. This learning is best done in small groups, being guided through a step-by-step program over the first two years of the course. In this way, simple practices become the basis from which more complex skills can develop. It is a steady, well-worked-out discipline, which needs to be established before students become able to work more fluidly as they near the end of their training.

Lying on a flat surface with the head supported and the knees bent allows the back to lengthen and widen and the breathing to deepen.

BACK LENGTHENS AND WIDENS

BREATHING DEEPENS

But in us they are special because they look this way

While our spine goes this way

PART TWO

The Use of the Self

PRACTICAL EXPERIENCE

ANATOMY AND PHYSIOLOGY

THE PROCEDURES

In us the spine goes UP

Look at the difference ...

The spine goes the same way as the eyes

and the eyes go FORWARD

THE USE OF THE SELF
PRACTICAL EXPERIENCE

LIKE PLANTS WE are living and growing, but unlike plants we are our own gardeners. We have conscious will, which gives us our overall direction. Gardening is not a random process, but involves making definite choices to avoid future problems. Alexander realized that how we maintain our upright posture represented a fundamental factor in the prevention of problems. There is no "correct" position to be held, for that which is right for you today cannot be the right one for tomorrow as you grow and develop. In life you are in a process of constant change. The Alexander Technique can help you cope with these changes. The possibility of growth and development only happens through change. We know this in our minds, but we have to make these changes in our bodies. There are no exercises in the Alexander Technique. There is no ideal posture to imitate and no hard and fast rules. You are finding a way of becoming more yourself.

Our bodies are gardens to the which our wills are gardeners so that if we plant nettles or sow lettuce, set hyssop and weed up thyme, supply it with one gender of herbs or distract it with many, either to have it sterile with idleness or manured with industry.

WILLIAM SHAKESPEARE: OTHELLO

USE AFFECTS FUNCTIONING

I prefer to call the psychophysical organism simply "the self" and to write of it as something "in use" which "functions" and "reacts."

F.M. ALEXANDER: THE UNIVERSAL CONSTANT IN LIVING

We use most things for a limited amount of time, then stop to go on to do something else. However, unlike tools and instruments our minds and bodies are in constant use. Most of the time we are not aware of this. As you use a kitchen knife, you are conscious of the knife and what you are cutting. Does it need sharpening? Is the handle getting a bit loose? Is it clean? Is it too near your fingers? You will be aware of the implement and its state. If it is not working well enough, you immediately try and fix it. Have you ever thought that you might need fixing? How are you holding the knife? Perhaps you are gripping it too tightly, or holding your breath as you chop, or tensing your shoulders, or bracing your knees? All of these will be affecting your level of efficiency and even wearing you out.

We do not drive our car in the way that we drive ourselves. If we use ourselves in a better way, we function more efficiently. Tension in the back muscles will shorten the spine, which normally bends the spine forward. There is a very simple experiment that you can try that makes it easy to see how the way you use something can increase or decrease its length. If you take a stick of a certain length and bend it, you will shorten the distance between both ends. If you bend yourself in such a way, you will shorten yourself by shortening and contracting your muscles. How your muscles operate affects your functioning. If you pull down, you will be squeezing your internal organs, holding onto your joints, restricting your breathing. All these may lead to problems and loss of vitality.

When you begin to pay attention to yourself, you can change how you use your mind and body, then your posture and physiology will change. The functioning of the circulatory system is changed, and as a consequence blood pressure is stabilized. Over the years we have gotten used to doing things habitually. We do not think about how we use ourselves. In order to change we have to pay more attention to our habits.

Young children display natural good use of the body as they have not formed any bad habits.

Short versus Tall

When you are neither collapsed nor trying to stand up too straight, your muscles and bones have a chance to achieve their full potential length. Compare gently holding a stick at both ends; the distance between both ends is not shortened.

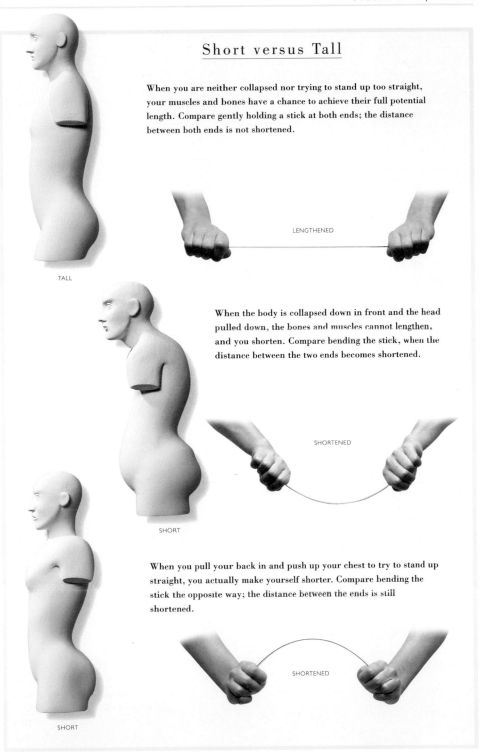

TALL

LENGTHENED

When the body is collapsed down in front and the head pulled down, the bones and muscles cannot lengthen, and you shorten. Compare bending the stick, when the distance between the two ends becomes shortened.

SHORT

SHORTENED

When you pull your back in and push up your chest to try to stand up straight, you actually make yourself shorter. Compare bending the stick the opposite way; the distance between the ends is still shortened.

SHORTENED

SHORT

HABITS

Of habits devil, is angel yet in this,
That aptly is put on. Refrain to-night;
And that shall lend a kind of easiness
To the next abstinence; the next more easy;
For use almost can change the
stamp of nature...

WILLIAM SHAKESPEARE: *HAMLET*

Habits are formed by repeating actions until they become settled, regular activities that are often hard to give up. When we first learn to do something, whether it is a basic skill like walking or a more refined complicated skill like playing an instrument or handling a tennis racket, we need to think about what we are doing. As we practice the skill, we still have to be conscious of what we are doing, but eventually it becomes automatic, a habit.

We may turn left on a journey because that is what we always do, although today we needed to turn right. In this way we become slaves to our habits, and it becomes more difficult to change as our lives change. Change can then become something difficult we have to do, instead of being exciting and inviting. In order to change a habit we have to go back to the time when we originally learned the skill. We have to change our

response from being unconscious of what we are doing to being more aware and conscious. We need to think about what we are doing. Have you ever gone to lift an empty box which you expected to be heavy? Often we generate far more effort than we need, and this imposes too much muscular tension on the body. It can become a vicious circle. Each time we use a certain amount of effort in an activity, like speaking, we will use it again because the effort becomes so closely associated with the act of speaking. When a habit is ingrained, it will feel as if we cannot speak unless we produce this effort. We need to have a way we can put this change into effect. The principles needed to break habits are conscious inhibition and conscious direction. We must reason out first what it is we want. In order to avoid employing the habit, we need to stop before we proceed.

Breaking Habits

If an attempt is to be made to change a person's habit, two things appear to be essential. The first is an adequate desire, on the part of the subject, to make the change. To achieve this, the helper needs to use his ingenuity to build up a suitable degree of motivation in the subject. The second requirement, and one which is much more difficult to meet, is that the person with the habit has to be brought to a condition in which he is aware of the "feel" of this changing condition which will, if allowed to proceed, eventually lead to the habitual movement. Once this crucial moment is recognized, he can take action to interpose an effective alternative pattern of behavior. From T.D.M. Roberts, *Understanding Balance*.

If I expect the box to be heavy, I make more effort than is necessary.

If I thought I had put sugar in my coffee but it was really salt... nasty surprise.

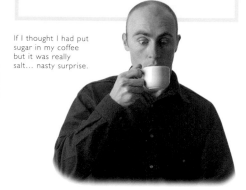

CONSCIOUS INHIBITION

*There is no evidence that inhibition is ever
accompanied by the slightest damage to the tissue;
on the contrary it seems to predispose the tissue
to a greater functional activity thereafter.*

SIR CHARLES SHERRINGTON

Inhibition is the practice of pausing before an action.
It gives us the time that is needed to register "how" we
are preparing for any activity and whether excessive
muscular tension is present. The inhibitory process
enables a release of the unnecessary contraction so that
the lengthening and widening of the body musculature
can be restored. Inhibition is a positive process,
leading to release, efficient preparation, and optimum
readiness. Why don't we think before we act? In *The
Use of the Self*, Alexander said:

*...I came to see at last that if I was ever to be able to
change my habitual use and dominate my instinctive
direction, it would be necessary for me to make the
experience of receiving the stimulus to speak and
refusing to do anything immediately in response.*

By stopping our habitual reactions, we give ourselves
a chance to stop rushing into things and a chance to
make a choice about how we do things. As our mental
attitude changes, there is a chance to break our habits.
Frank Pierce Jones said in *Freedom to Change*:

*Inhibition is a positive, not a negative
force. Some degree of inhibition is
essential not only for a good life
but for any life at all...
Inhibition is a physiological
process which does not need to
be conscious in order to
operate. Bringing it up to the
conscious level not only
establishes an indirect
control over anti-gravity*

*See a good habit
makes a child a man
Whereas a bad one
makes a man a beast.*

JOHN WEBSTER: *THE WHITE DEVIL*

Experiment with mirror

Try this experiment. Stand in front of a
mirror and decide to speak. What do you
do? Do you react and stiffen your neck, brace
your legs, hold your breath? Take a second to
say "No" to those habits that upset your poise
and calmness. Free your neck, let your head go
forward and up, let your back lengthen and
widen, and breathe out before you speak. Do
you notice any differences especially in the
sound of your voice?

*responses but facilitates the learning of new
habits and the unlearning of those that are old
and unwanted. When a stimulus is presented for
the first time, many responses are available,
including not making a response at all. If one of
these responses is selected and learned, it can be
repeated without loss of choice as long as the
process remains conscious. If it drops below the
level of consciousness, a "set" will be established
linking the stimulus with the response, which will
then occur automatically whether it is
appropriate or not... The result is a
habit which operates unconsciously
(like an innate reflex) and which is
resistant to change. Inhibition
raises the level of tonic activity in
the nervous system, brings the
operation of the habit to a
conscious level, and restores choice
(including the choice of making the
original response).*

*For the good that I would
I do not,
But the evil which I would not,
that I do.*

ROMANS 7:19

CONSCIOUS DIRECTION

JACK: "You're quite perfect, Miss Fairfax."
GWENDOLEN: "Oh! I hope I am not that.
It would leave no room for
developments, and I intend to
develop in many directions."

OSCAR WILDE:
THE IMPORTANCE OF BEING EARNEST

All the time in life, we are giving ourselves directions. We have conversations with ourselves about what we want to happen. "Smarten up, pull yourself together, get real, try hard, don't give up, get your act together, don't go wrong." We can give ourselves these instructions to find our way, as we follow directions on a map. As we map-read, we work out where we are and in which direction we need to go. Always we are going from here to there. When we are lost, we are grateful for any information that is clearly and confidently given – turn left after the lights, keep right on to the end of the road, then take the first

OSCAR WILDE
1854–1900

left. In the same way we can work out where we are and in which direction we need to go. Alexander observed that certain directions are not as helpful as others. We cannot see directions, but we can see the result of them in the posture and form of our ourselves. Alexander formulated the directions "Let the neck be free so that the head can go forward and up so that the back can lengthen and widen" to give himself a clear route to follow.

Conscious directions are instructions given to enable the body to release, lengthen, and widen. It is by giving conscious directions that we encourage our bodies to adopt their full stature. Direction does not involve a direct command; rather it is a process of giving suggestions that encourage a reflex process to happen and avoid interference with the natural poise of our upright posture.

There exists in these directions an implicit message that we have to give ourselves time for this to happen. These directions can enable us to come back to the shape that nature intended. If we have no directions or choose not to follow them, then we could get lost.

HEAD GOES
FORWARD AND UP

NECK IS FREE

BACK LENGTHENS
AND WIDENS

Direction

As an animal walks forward, the head is in a direct horizontal line with the spine. The movement of the head goes in the same direction as the movement of the body. The head acts as a balancer, regulating the weight carried by the front and hind legs as it is lowered or raised, usually toward food.

END-GAINING AND MEANS-WHEREBY

In the 1930s Aldous Huxley had lessons from Alexander from which he benefited tremendously. He believed that the Alexander Technique was unique in its ability to deal with the problem of "end-gaining." "End-gaining" describes the process in which a person is preoccupied with goals and disregards how the goals are attained – the means-whereby. At worst, "end-gaining" advocates the end at any cost, an obsession with outcomes with no regard to the cost to the psycho-physical organism. Huxley (quoted in Frank Pierce Jones, *Freedom to Change*) said:

DON'T TRY
TOO HARD

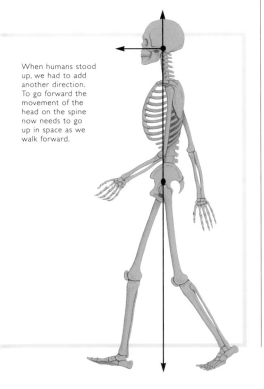

One has to make the discovery for oneself, starting from scratch and to find what old F.M. Alexander called "the means-whereby," without which good intentions merely pave hell, and the idealist remains an ineffectual, self-destructive and other-destructive end-gainer.

When humans stood up, we had to add another direction. To go forward the movement of the head on the spine now needs to go up in space as we walk forward.

Aldous Huxley

Aldous Huxley (1894–1963) was an English novelist and essayist. In *Brave New World* (1932) he warns of the dangers of moral anarchy in a scientific age. He said in 1944 in *Time must have a Stop* that "There's only one corner of the universe you can be certain of improving, and that's your own self."

The Alexander Technique encourages you to observe and think about how you work to gain your end. The basic learning skills that any child develops rely on this way of learning. The child is told to think about what he is doing, to take his time, to take care, and not to panic. These instructions are the "means-whereby" the child gains his ends. When not enough attention is paid to how that end is gained, problems can arise. Have you ever found that the harder you try, the more difficult it is to achieve your goals? Let me give you an example:

If you perform breathing exercises in order to have a greater lung capacity, you could be actually creating more tensions in your body and undermining your inherent potential to breathe naturally, fully, and freely. Because you are concentrating on the exercise of breathing and trying too hard to achieve results too quickly, you will be defeating yourself. When you "end-gain," you can block results because you generate excessive muscular tension in your determination to get what you want.

Often it seems to us that our day consists of a long list of activities, things we have to get done. We rush through these tasks as quickly as possible with the thought of enjoying ourselves afterward. We end up not enjoying our daily activities because they have become unpleasant tasks. Often they have become unpleasant activities because of the excessive muscular tension we have created as we rush to try to get them over and done with. It is a vicious circle that can be broken by attending to the means whereby we gain our ends. The Alexander Technique enables us to develop the sensitivity that gives us a more accurate perception of ourselves and how we do things. We strive to be "on time," fearful of being late and tend to forget that we also need to be "in time" and "in tune."

35

SENSORY APPRECIATION: THE SEARCHLIGHT OF ATTENTION

We are familiar with our five senses: taste, touch, sight, smell, hearing. Sensory appreciation is our conscious evaluation of these senses. Perhaps you have never realized that you have a sixth sense, proprioception. This is the ability to understand and use the signals that your balance mechanism and movement receptors send to your brain.

A lot of the time we are unaware that we have this sense. We do not feel quite right. Like Hamlet we feel, "like sweet bells, jangled and out of tune." We are unaware of ourselves. Have you ever been surprised by a photograph of yourself – "I don't look like that! I didn't realize I was doing that!" Have you caught a reflection of yourself in a window and been surprised at how you are standing?

When you look in a mirror, you can see what you are doing. This can cause quite a shock – back hollowed, head pulled back, knees locked. As you change to a "better" posture, the new one can look and feel wrong to you. You are used to your old body position, so the new posture pattern seems strange. It takes time to adopt a new posture, even though the benefits are obvious both visually and in your physiological functioning and general well-being. Dr. G.E. Coghill in the Appreciation for *The Universal Constant in Living*, said:

> *Alexander has further demonstrated the very important psychological principle that the proprioceptive system can be brought under conscious control and can be educated to carry to the motor centers the stimulus that is responsible for the muscular activity that brings about the manner of working (use) of the mechanism of correct posture.*

SMELL

TOUCH

HEARING

TASTE

SIGHT

SIXTH SENSE

We see, we hear, we smell, we touch, we taste, but it is our sixth sense, our sensory appreciation, that lets us evaluate the other five senses.

Her pure and eloquent blood
Spoke in her cheeks, and so distinctly wrought
That one might almost say, her body thought.
JOHN DONNE: *OF THE PROGRESS OF THE SOUL*
(*SECOND ANNIVERSARY*: 1612).

THE ALEXANDER TECHNIQUE BRINGS YOU TO YOUR SENSES

Alexander showed that it is possible to be unaware of what we are doing. It is generally assumed that feelings give us accurate information about our body. When this feedback is incorrect, our sensory appreciation becomes unreliable. In connection with unreliable sensory appreciation the following story was related by Alexander in *Constructive Conscious Control*:

A little girl who had been unable to walk properly for some years was brought to the writer for a diagnosis of the defects in the use of the psychophysical mechanisms that were responsible for her more or less crippled state. When this had been done, a request was made that a demonstration should be given to those present of the manipulative side of the work so that certain readjustments and coordinations might be temporally secured, thus showing, in keeping with the diagnosis, the possibilities of re-education on a general basis in a case of this kind. The demonstration was successful from this point of view. For the time being, the child's body was comparatively straightened out – that is, without the extreme twists and distortions that had been so noticeable when she came into the room. When this was done, the little girl looked across at her mother and said to her in indescribable tone, "Oh, Mommy, he has pulled me all out of shape." Her deceptive feelings led this little girl to believe that she was standing straight, when she was all out of shape. We are often under the same misconception. What we do feels right because it is our habitual way of acting, no matter how wrong and unsatisfactory it is in reality.

Change involves carrying out an activity against the habits of a lifetime. This is one of the most challenging aspects of practicing the Alexander Technique, but the reward is a more finely tuned perception.

Proprioception

Proprioception is a term first used by the eminent neurophysiologist Sir Charles Sherrington. It is our secret sixth sense. It is the process through which human beings get information from their bodies, ascertain their position in space, and recognize whether too much muscular effort is being used. This instinctive and unconscious process has developed and acted as a trustworthy guide throughout the course of evolution, ensuring correct and efficient posture and ease in movement. Sensory appreciation allows us to consciously receive and evaluate this information and lets us know whether our body is functioning well. Refined sensory appreciation improves the feedback from all the senses.

The martial arts require a high degree of sensory appreciation and control of the musculature.

Kirlian photography captures our proprioceptive energy on film.

PRIMARY CONTROL

There is a primary control of the use of the self which governs the working of all the mechanisms and so renders the control of the complex human organism comparatively simple.

F.M. ALEXANDER: *THE USE OF THE SELF*

Everybody who has a head, neck, and back has a primary control. Children and animals move with co-ordinated grace, because they allow this facility to inform all movement. Primary control consists of the processes that control the use of the head and neck in relation to the back. It is primary because it comes first in every movement. To a large extent it determines the coordination and muscle tones of the rest of the body. The parts of the body should be used in harmony with the primary control, that coordinated action of the head, neck, and back working together, creating a total pattern of use. Alexander discovered, by observing his movements through the feedback the mirror gave him, that he habitually interfered with his head–neck–back relationship.

That the neck is of great importance for the control of balance and posture in animals has been known since

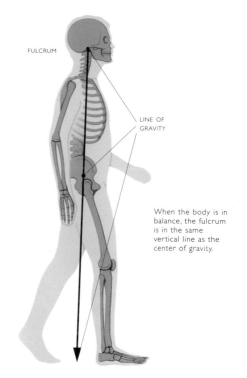

FULCRUM

LINE OF GRAVITY

When the body is in balance, the fulcrum is in the same vertical line as the center of gravity.

Daniel Pevsner and his horse provide an excellent display of primary control.

Balance

Poise and balance are not fixed but fully mobile. When you come to measure something on a balance scale, first of all check that the pivot is free. Put the scales down and see whether they are set to measure efficiently by checking that the horizontal beam is parallel. If it is not, then anything you put in the pans to weigh will not be measured accurately. Compare this with how you check your own head balance.

is back and down, the body weight forward, and the spine shortened, a stooped posture is created. The delicate balance of the head on the neck can be upset quite easily. Sensory input from the neck muscles is very important physiologically. The number of nerve receptors in neck muscles is much higher than in other muscles. The control of muscles in posture and movement is primarily affected by the state of neck muscles with their very strong sensory input to the brain.

The procedures used in the Alexander Technique help to establish a new dynamic balance among the forces acting on the head, so that more of the postural work can be done by disks, ligaments, and muscles acting at their optimal length. The head feels lighter because more of its weight is carried by muscles that have lengthened. The increase in the axis of head rotation facilitates extension of the spine in all movements. The space between all the vertebrae and especially between the first vertebra and the head increases, creating more room for blood vessels so that more blood flows to the brain. This improves all mental and physical activities.

the 19th century when vivisectionists showed that cutting the posterior neck muscles resulted in severe disturbances of posture and locomotion in animals.

When the head is forward and up, the weight of the body is back, the spine lengthened, and a balanced upright posture results. When the head

Primary Control

Question: What does the Primary Control control?

Answer: The dynamic relationship between the head, neck, and torso that maintains the balance and preempts falling or collapse.

Question: Who exercises this Primary Control?

Answer: You do!

OUT OF BALANCE

HEAD FREELY BALANCED ON SPINE

When the relationship between the head, neck, and spine is correct, any activity is improved.

ANATOMY: THE STRUCTURE

WHAT DETERMINES OUR shape? Growth patterns, genetic endowment, environment, education, training, life experiences, trauma, success, potential – tapped, untapped. We are changing position all the time, so our shape is constantly changing. Shape is roughly determined by bones and muscles. Bone is a living substance, capable of great changes, including degeneration. Muscles can adopt very different shapes and maintain them through constant use and misuse.

He has lost connection with the Head, from whom the whole body, supported and held together by its ligaments and sinews grows as God causes it to grow.

COLOSSIANS 2: 19

All muscles in animals, including humans, are in a state of mild contraction even when seemingly still. Maintaining a static (unmoving) posture demands muscular activity just as any movement does. Just to stand, the muscles which oppose one another on either side of the knee, hip, and ankle must exert an equal and opposite tension. This stabilizes the joints and prevents them from collapsing under the body's weight. Movement is simply the change from one stance to the next. When you move one of your limbs, you increase the state of contraction on one side of the joint and decrease a proportional amount on the other side. When a "good" posture is adopted, it means that the contractions of the muscles are adequate to maintain the body in such a way that favors the best functioning and puts minimal strain on the muscles, tendons, ligaments, and bones. The reverse is true of the effects of "bad" posture. Besides the obvious detraction from appearance, poor posture makes you tire more quickly. Abnormal pulls are put on tendons, ligaments, joints, and bones, and can lead to deformities. Poor posture decreases the breathing capacity of the lungs. Posture directly affects your bodily functions. We often associate good posture with being straight and poor posture with being bent. However, there is nothing straight in the human body. Everything is designed on the principle of curves. These curves are developed as a baby learns to hold up its head and stand, and provide balance in the upright position. *(Refer to the section "Growth and Development of Children," page 98.)* They give strength to support the weight of the rest of the body. A curved structure has more strength than a straight one made of the same material of the same size.

The dictionary defines man as "an individual of the highest type of animal existing, especially in his extraordinary mental development." The Latin name for man is *Homo sapiens* – translated as the Thinking Man.

Muscle Control

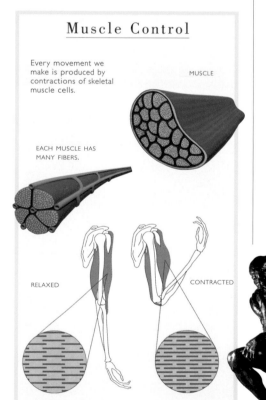

Every movement we make is produced by contractions of skeletal muscle cells.

MUSCLE

EACH MUSCLE HAS MANY FIBERS.

RELAXED

CONTRACTED

THE SKELETAL SYSTEM

The skeleton provides support for the body and gives protection to the delicate organs. It serves to provide points of attachment for the muscles in such a way that the bones can function with the muscles as a lever system. The bones of the skeleton also manufacture blood cells and act as storehouses for minerals.

THE AXIAL SKELETON

The bones of the skull, spine, and chest, and the hyoid bone in the neck, make up the axial skeleton.

The axial skeleton is colored red in this illustration, and the appendicular skeleton is colored blue.

SKULL

HYOID BONE

CHEST

SPINE

The Skull

The skull is made up of 28 bones. Eight of these form the cranium, 14 form the face, and six form the middle ear. These bones protect the brain and also carry and protect the important sense organs of the eyes, ears, and nose.

The skull is not solid bone, which would be impossibly heavy, but has sinuses, which are spaces inside the cranium. The bone at the base of the skull (occiput) makes a joint with the top vertebra of the spinal column (atlas), which allows the head pivotal movement between the first and the second vertebrae (axis). This joint is called the atlantooccipital joint and enables the skull to nod, which is crucial to the freedom of our upright posture and our entire movement pattern. The spinal cord enters the cranium through a large hole (foranum magnum) in the occipital bone. The upper jaw (maxilla) is part of the skull, but the lower jaw is hinged for movement by a condyloid joint that permits all types of movement except rotation, including opening, closing, sliding, chewing, crushing.

The Vertebrae (Spinal Column)

The spinal column needs to meet two contradictory mechanical requirements – stability and mobility. It consists of 24 individual vertebrae made up of bone, with a channel in the middle through which the spinal cord, a bundle of nerve pathways running from the brain, passes. In this position the cord is protected from damage. Each vertebra is separated from the next one by an intervertebral disk made of fibrous cartilage that acts as a shock-absorbing cushion. These disks conform to the size of the vertebrae. They not only absorb any shock that may be delivered to the spinal column, but also aid in its mobility.

TRANSVERSE PROCESS

TRANSVERSE PROCESS

BODY

SPINAL CANAL

BODY

The Breastbone and Ribs

The breastbone (sternum) is shaped like a dagger, with the bone ending with a piece of cartilage called the xiphoid process. It forms the point of articulation for the collarbone (clavicle) and is the anterior attachment point for the ribs. The ribs

RIBS AND STERNUM

1–10 are anchored to the 12 thoracic vertebrae, but ribs 11 and 12, floating ribs, are not attached to the front. The bone of the rib is called the shaft and is somewhat flattened. The lower border of the shaft has a costal groove that protects the blood vessels and nerves that course along each rib.

These 12 pairs of ribs form a bony cage known as the chest (or thorax). The rib cage is shaped like a barrel with ribs 1–7 getting larger, then 7–12 getting progressively smaller. The lungs lie enclosed within an airtight thoracic cavity. The structure of the chest cavity is such that its volume can be made to increase or decrease. The skeletal framework is almost completely filled with lungs and heart. The dimensions of the thoracic cavity can increase in three planes during inhalation.

Cartilage

Cartilage or gristle is a smooth tough tissue that varies throughout the skeleton, according to the special job it has to do. Hyaline cartilage is the most ridged of the three and is found in the cartilage of the joints, the costal (rib) cartilage, the nose, larynx (voice box), trachea (windpipe), and bronchi (branches of the trachea). Laryngeal cartilage controls the amount of air passing through the larynx, which determines the pitch of the note.

Osteoporosis

Osteoporosis is one of the most common and serious of all bone diseases. The bone degenerates, and the incidence of "spontaneous fractures" can increase. Although some bone loss is an accepted consequence of advancing years, the effects of osteoporosis on the spine are abnormal. In addition to the common treatment of sex hormone therapy and dietary supplements of calcium and vitamin D, physical activity may play a part in minimizing degeneration.

THE APPENDICULAR SKELETON

The limbs are movable appendages. There are 126 bones in the appendicular skeleton, which consists of the bones of the upper and lower extremities and of the pectoral girdle and the pelvic girdle.

Bones of the Upper Extremities

The shoulder girdle (pectoral girdle) includes the clavicle and scapula (shoulder blade) and with the arms, wrists, and hands comprises the bones of the upper extremities. The clavicle is essentially a strut that projects the scapula far enough laterally to clear the barrel-shaped chest wall. The scapula carries the arm and is a thin, flat, triangular plate of bone covered with muscles on both sides. It lies freely movable on the posterior–superior wall of the rib cage.

The upper appendicular skeleton consists of the bones of the shoulders, pectoral girdles, arms, and hands.

ULNA
RADIUS
CARPALS
METACARPALS
PHALANGES

The Arm

Attached to the scapula at its proximal end is the long upper bone of the arm (humerus). Long bones are cylinders of hard bone with soft marrow on the inside.

The upper arm articulates with the two bones (radius and ulna) of the lower arm (forearm) at the elbow joint. The radius is the bone on the thumb side of the lower arm, the ulna is the bone on the little finger side of the lower arm. The elbow is a combined joint. A hinged joint connects the humerus and ulna, and a ball-and-socket joint connects the ulna to the radius, surrounded by synovial membrane, a thin sheet of tissue that allows for freer movement with less friction. This combined joint allows the arm to bend at the elbow and turns the palm upward and downward.

HUMERUS

The elbow is a combined hinge and ball-and-socket joint, allowing rotational as well as lateral movement.

Hands and Wrist

The wrists and hands have more bones for their size than any other part of the body, 27 bones in all. The tips of the fingers can touch any point in the three-dimensional sphere. The hand is capable of highly complex movements. It gives us the possibility to grip things and carry out delicate complicated movements that require a high degree of coordination, for example, writing. *(See the section "Handwriting," page 70.)* The dexterity of our hand movements is one of the distinguishing features of human evolution. Prehension is the essential function of the hand. The thumb can come into contact with each finger. This special movement is called opposition. The hand also gives feedback about thickness and distance to the brain, allowing for the development of visual appreciation.

Bones of the Lower Extremities

Two hip bones and the sacrum link to form the pelvic girdle. The long bone of the thigh (femur) forms a deep ball-and-socket joint with the hip bone. The femur articulates with the shin bone (tibia) to form the knee joint. The knee is the intermediate joint of the lower limb. It needs to have great stability and mobility. It is beautifully designed for these two things, but is liable to strains and dislocations. A long slender bone (fibula) lies alongside the tibia, and together they form the top of the ankle joint.

HIP BONES

FEMUR

PATELLA

FIBULA

TIBIA

TARSALS

METATARSALS

The lower appendicular skeleton consists of the bones of the hips, pelvic girdle, legs, ankles, and feet.

The Foot

There are seven tarsal bones in each foot, which form the heel, back of the foot, and the bottom of the ankle joint, and articulate with five metatarsals, which form the midfoot to which the toes are attached. There are 14 toe bones (phalanges), three in each of the smaller toes and two in each big toe.

The foot needs to be able to support the body's weight, so the bony design forms an arched structure that is reinforced with strong ligaments, allowing for shock absorption and spring in locomotion. Strong ligaments and leg muscle tendons normally hold the foot bones firmly in position. However, if the foot tendons or ligaments weaken, the arches flatten and fallen arches or flat feet result.

Joints

Joints are classified anatomically into two types, mobile or synovial joints, and fixed or fibrous joints. Synovial joints are designed to allow a large range of movements and are lined with a slippery coating called synovium. Fibrous joint movement is limited by fibrous tissue.

Fibrous (spine)

Synovial (hinge)

HOW DOES IT ALL LINK UP?

Every bone in the body (with the exception of the hyoid bone which is part of the suspensory mechanism of the larynx) connects to at least one other bone by a joint. Joints hold the bones together and make movement possible. There would be no way of moving the arms or legs or any other part of the body without joints.

Skeletal Muscle

Skeletal muscle is responsible for body movements, maintaining our upright posture, and generating body heat. Skeletal muscles are like springs attached to the skeleton at various points throughout the body. Their main function is to connect bone to bone over a movable joint. They make up a large proportion of our body weight. The sustained constriction of skeletal muscle can distort our natural posture over time and interfere with the ability to lengthen and widen in stature. Skeletal muscle is activated by messages sent voluntarily to the motor nerves in the spinal cord. As the signal is received, the muscle shortens as the fibers contract, and this moves the bone.

Muscle tissue, popularly called flesh, accounts for about 40 percent of our body weight. The muscular system plays a vital role in healthy living. In the human body, movement occurs as the muscles contract and shorten. They achieve this by converting chemical energy obtained from food into mechanical energy that then pulls on the bones and moves them. To do this the muscle is first stimulated by nerve impulses. Individual muscles can act only to shorten the distance between attachment points – they can pull but not push. For movement in the opposite direction to occur, another muscle must be activated. This action is called "antagonistic," which means "working against each other," and the muscles that work in this way are called antagonists.

Each muscle has many muscle fibers, bundled together in an envelope of connective tissue. A small muscle may consist of only a few bundles of fibers, while a large muscle like the buttock (gluteus maximus) has hundreds of bundles.

Muscles

There are three different types of muscles in the body. Together with the bones and tendons, they are responsible for movement.

SKELETAL MUSCLE (voluntary striated muscle) This muscle is attached to the bones.

VISCERAL MUSCLE (involuntary smooth muscle) This muscle forms the walls of the blood vessels and the hollow internal organs – the viscera, including the gut (stomach and intestines), and the bronchial tubes.

CARDIAC MUSCLE (involuntary muscle) This muscle forms the bulk of the heart.

TRAPEZIUS

PECTORALIS MAJOR

RECTUS ABDOMINUS

GLUTEUS MAXIMUS

QUADRICEPS

HAMSTRINGS

The active body of the muscle is attached to tendons that join onto the bone (see Tendons below). The bone is pulled across movable joints. The muscle that is predominantly responsible for a particular movement is called the prime mover. The muscles that help in that movement are called synergists. Muscles do not function alone and depend on the functioning of other parts of the body.

Tendons

Tendons anchor muscles to bones and also link muscles to muscles. They are very strong and are made of dense, fibrous connective tissue, which is non-elastic. Some tendons are enclosed in sheaths, which are tubelike structures lubricated by synovial fluid, which allow easier body movement.

Bursae are small fluid-filled sacs that lie between some tendons and the bones beneath them. They are lined with synovial membrane, which secretes the slippery, lubricating synovial fluid that fills each bursa. They act as cushions against severe stress and make for easier movement of the tendons sliding over the bones. Both tendons and bursae are subject to inflammation (see Box).

If muscle cells are stimulated repeatedly without adequate periods of rest, the strength of muscle contraction decreases, resulting in fatigue.

Tendonitis and Tenosynovitis

Tendonitis and tenosynovitis are painful conditions caused by the tendon or the sheath of the tendon becoming inflamed. The problem commonly occurs in wrists, fingers, and forearms. Activities such as racket sports, which demand repetitive movements of the wrists, or typing and word processing, which demand repetitive finger movements, are liable to produce this condition. It is popularly known as Repetitive Strain Injury (R.S.I.), and the number of sufferers is steadily increasing. The *British Medical Journal* now refers to this as work-related upper limb disorder. Reducing the stress on muscles, tendons, and joints can help relieve and prevent these debilitating conditions.

Head Retraction

When the muscles of the neck shorten and pull the head back and down, or hold it in a fixed position, neck aches and headaches can result. This also has an adverse effect on the rest of the body, because of the increased strain and extra weight.

THE BREATHING MECHANISM

The breathing mechanism consists primarily of the skeleton and muscles of the torso, which divides into the upper cavity (chest/thoracic cavity) and the lower cavity (abdomen). The chest cavity is filled almost completely by the lungs and heart, and the abdomen with the digestive tract, glands, and vital organs (viscera). Breathing is controlled by the respiratory control centers in the medulla, the hindmost segment of the brain. Under resting conditions, nervous activity in the respiratory control centers (R.C.C.s) produces a normal state and depth of breathing (12–18 respirations per minute) and in 24 hours we shift 1,850 gallons of air. The R.C.C.s are influenced by inputs from receptors located in other body areas. The cerebral cortex, the outer gray matter of the brain, can influence respiration by modifying the rate at which the nerves (neurones) "fire" in the R.C.C. In other words, you can change your breathing pattern during activities such as speaking, eating, and swimming, when you are able to hold your breath for short periods. This voluntary control has definite limits.

The contraction of the diaphragm makes the chest cavity longer from top to bottom. As we breathe in the diaphragm, the large sheet of muscle shaped like a dome, which separates the thorax and the abdomen, contracts and is drawn down into the abdomen. This increases the chest cavity and the volume of the air

The regular practice of comfortable rhythmic breathing as part of a good swimming style strengthens our breathing mechanism.

in the lungs. Once in the lungs, air travels to the alveoli, the terminal air sacs of the lungs, where oxygen is taken up by the blood cells, and CO_2 is discharged. As we breathe out, the diaphragm is drawn upward into the chest cavity, and the volume of air in the lungs decreases. Overcontraction of the muscles of the chest restricts the movement of the ribcage.

When the muscles of the rib cage (external intercostal muscles) contract, they enlarge the chest cavity by increasing its size from front to back and from side to side, and air is drawn into the lungs. During more forceful expiration (speaking, singing, heavy work, lifting), the internal intercostal muscles and the abdominal muscles contract and the chest cavity decreases in size from top to bottom, and air flows out of the lungs.

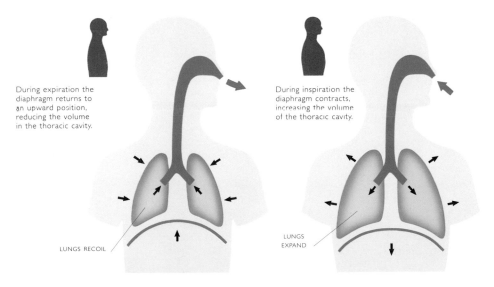

During expiration the diaphragm returns to an upward position, reducing the volume in the thoracic cavity.

LUNGS RECOIL

During inspiration the diaphragm contracts, increasing the volume of the thoracic cavity.

LUNGS EXPAND

PHYSIOLOGY: HOW IT WORKS

HUMANS HAVE A greater variety of mobility and a greater versatility of movement than animals. To move, we need energy. The Alexander Technique believes that this energy must be correctly directed. The more energy you have, the more potential damage you can do to both yourself and other persons and things.

GRAVITY AND WEIGHT

Although we have become accustomed to using scales to measure weight, weight is actually a variable matter of gravity working on the body.

Remember the momentary feeling of weightlessness when a plane hits an air pocket? You feel as if you have left your seat. Or the feeling of your stomach staying behind you as you go up in a fast elevator? For a constant weight measurement, we need constant conditions.

The gravitational attraction of the Earth pulls every particle of the body down toward the Earth's center. At the same time, the body mass attracts every particle of the Earth, giving a resultant upward force on the earth and acting through its center. These two gravitational forces are both equal and opposite. The downward force on the body corresponds to the force responsible for the curvature of the path of unsupported objects and for the curvature of orbits. The upward force on the Earth corresponds to the action of the moon in raising the tide.

Gravity allows us to stand on the ground and relate
to the Earth. It is our way of knowing stability.
Where do we stand, and how do we deal with space?

TESSA MARWICK,
DIRECTOR OF ALEXANDER TECHNIEK CENTRUM, AMSTERDAM

Why, man, he doth bestride the
narrow world like a Colossus
WILLIAM SHAKESPEARE: *JULIUS CAESAR*

WEIGHT IS THE STRESS FORCE WITH WHICH AN OBJECT PRESSES DOWN ON ITS SUPPORTS.

When an object is at rest on the Earth's surface, its supports exert a stress force at the area of contact.

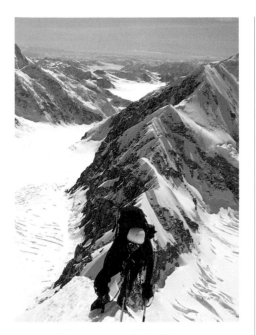

I live not in myself, but I become
Portion of that around me; and to me
High mountains are a feeling.
BYRON: *CHILDE HAROLD'S PILGRIMAGE*

Professor T. D. M. Roberts is a leading authority in the neurophysiology of posture. In his book *The Neurophysiology of the Postural Mechanisms* (1967), he argues that the primary aim of the neuromuscular mechanism is to counteract the downward force of gravity. He identifies the postural reflexes as forces working to thrust the body into space, mechanisms designed to counteract the downward force of gravity with minimal effort and in such a way that we are able to realize our full physiological stature with ease and freedom: he says that the primary requirement of the neuromuscular mechanism is to make sure the head does not come into punishing collisions with its environment. The mechanism ensures that it avoids this collision by generating anticipatory preemptive actions. This means that the mechanism is anticipating and forecasting on the basis of messages received through the kinesthetic/proprioceptive network, whether or not the self, i.e. the head and body, is in danger of falling down, and preempts that by generating up-thrusting movements that counteract and rescue the self from the downward influence of gravity.

FRANK PIERCE JONES
Author of Freedom to Change

My strongest impression when A.R. Alexander first demonstrated the Technique to me was that of a mechanism working against gravity. I could not see what Alexander's brother had done, but I could perceive its effect on me. I was occupying more space; my movements were less jerky; and I had lost my customary feeling of heaviness. Whatever his procedures were, they had made a radical change in my relation to the gravitational field. The change was not an illusion, since the sensory effect lasted for the rest of the day. It was a new experience that I had neither learned nor willed. There must, I thought, be a mechanism or set of mechanisms already present – a physiological a priori, to use Magnus's term – to account for the effect.

In its relations with human beings, gravity has generally had a bad name. It is commonly thought of as a hostile force that has to be fought against and overcome. One of the most eloquent expressions of this feeling about gravity was made by the biologist D'Arcy W. Thompson. In his great book *On Growth and Form* he wrote:

Man's slow decline in stature is a sign of the unequal contest between our bodily powers and the unchanging force of gravity which draws us down when we would fain rise up. We strive against it all our days, in every movement of our limbs, in every beat of our hearts. Gravity makes a difference to a man's height, and no slight one, between the morning and the evening; it leaves its mark in sagging wrinkles, drooping mouth and hanging breasts; it is the indomitable force which defeats us in the end, which lays us on our death bed and lowers us to the grave.

SPIRALS

One of the basic principles upon which matter and energy are organized is spirals. Growth patterns in plants, whirlpools, whirlwinds, and the spiral galaxies are all based on spiral movements. Human anatomy reflects these universal principles. Think of throwing a ball or a discus. There is an upward thrust in the whole body that allows the arm to come around and hurl the object. This spiral spring is important in nature. Human anatomy reflects these universal principles; nothing is completely straight. All the bones, joints, and muscle structures are spirally formed. Even the structure of the heart is built on this spiral pattern. When you watch someone curl up for a sleep, the spirals are working beautifully. Conversely, when someone gets themself "all in a twist," you see the whole body pulling in a whirlpool of tension.

Galaxies are cosmic examples of spirals.

Thinking the instruction "Let the neck be free so the head can go forward and up and the back can lengthen and widen" allows the deep spirals that connect the head to the hips to release.

How Directions and Spirals Relate

Spirals run from either side of the base of the skull. They cross the spine at the shoulder-blades and follow the ribs around to the front. Then they cross the abdomen diagonally to attach to the top of the pelvic crest.

Thinking the instruction "let your knees go forward and away" allows the two spirals connecting the legs to the torso to release. The first spiral runs from the arch of the foot, up the inner calf, through the knee to the outer thigh, around the buttocks to the sacrum and the back crest of the pelvis. The second spiral runs from the outer edge and top of the foot, up the outer calf, around the knee, and up the inner thigh over the front of the pelvis to attach to the front of the lumbar spine.

Thinking about the direction of widening across the upper part of the body allows the two spirals of the arm to release. The first spiral runs from the thumb and palm, up the inside of the forearm through the elbow to the back of the upper arm, then fans out from the shoulder to the head and upper back (trapezius). The second spiral runs from the little finger through the back of the hand to the back of the forearm, then through the inner upper arm to the armpit, after which it fans out and down to the lower back and sacrum.

REFLEXES

Sherrington wrote extensively on the relationship between reflex, muscular control, and conscious volition. The most well-known clinical reflex is the knee-jerk. He proved that in the muscles were sensitive muscle spindles that were linked to the spinal cord via nerve fibers. It was the muscle spindles sending a shower of sensory impulses into the spinal cord that caused the reflex. He observed that for every action there was an equal and opposite inhibition of the action of the muscle, which would normally be its mechanical opponent. In order to allow the muscle in the front of the thigh to shorten, the muscle in the back of the thigh lengthens.

The word "reflex" is used to denote any rapid action, including the highly skilled reactions of competitive athletes.

Any act...which employs a (voluntary) muscle cannot fail to enlist reflex action from it... This reflex factor is as important for the right performance of movement and posture as is the tuning of a string for the harmonious use of it in music.

Alexander said that "we do not know how we use ourselves any more than a dog or a cat knows." When it comes to physical coordination, none of us knows what we are doing. If we did, we probably wouldn't be able to do it. When Alexander said, "the right thing does itself," he was referring to a reflex process that must not be interfered with, and must not be controlled if it is going to be able to "do itself." Sherrington believed that:

This mastery of the brain over the reflex machinery does not take the form of intermeddling with reflex details; rather it dictates to a reflex mechanism "you may act" or "you may not act."

The functioning of a specific movement reflects the overall functioning of the organism. Sherrington paid tribute to Alexander's practical treatment of this issue when he said:

In urbanized and industrialized communities, bad habits in our motor acts are especially common. But verbal instruction as to how to correct wrong habits of movement and posture is very difficult. The scantiness of our sensory perception of how we do them makes it so... Mr. Alexander has done a service to the subject by insistently treating each act as involving the whole integrated individual, the whole psychophysical man. To take a step is an affair, not of this or that limb solely, but of the total neuromuscular activity of the moment – not least of the head and neck.

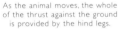

As the animal moves, the whole of the thrust against the ground is provided by the hind legs.

MUSCLE FIBER

Muscle fibers divide into white fibers for strength and red fibers for rhythmic movement and posture. Red fibers (postural fibers), though not as strong as white fibers, do not tire as quickly and are therefore ideally suited for maintaining the appropriate curve of the lower back which allows lengthening to take place.

When inadequate use is made of postural fibers, notably the deeper paraspinal muscles, then problems of posture arise. An extreme example is the experience of astronauts who, despite exercising to maintain the endurance and strength of their muscles in space, experience some atrophy that seems predominantly to affect the red fibers. Experiments with rats indicate that, following a period of time in space, their white muscle

Reduced Gravity

Humans can lose the use of their postural fibers as a result of not using them appropriately to deal with gravity. If a person habitually overcontracts their muscles to stand upright or constantly adopts a collapsed posture, then the red postural fibers atrophy because they are not being used and become less able to support the back efficiently. From Dr. David Garlick's discussion, the following suggestions can be made regarding muscle function:

1. The force of gravity is essential to activate the red postural fibers – if you do not have gravity, the red fibers deteriorate.

2. Red muscle fibers can either atrophy or go through a conversion where they become like white fibers.

3. When red fibers have atrophied or changed to white fibers, they lose their ability to act as muscles of posture.

4. The deep muscles of the back that are concerned with posture are controlled at a subconscious level and work by reflexes.

POISED

WEIGHED
DOWN

African women of certain tribes can move heavy loads freely by using the body as a pendulum during locomotion.

fibers were virtually unchanged, but the red fibers of their back showed both atrophy and a change in their characteristics, by which they became more like white fibers. The force of gravity is necessary for the postural fibers to be stimulated.

Dr. David Garlick explains that:

the red postural fibers, particularly of back muscles used to support the trunk, require tonic (that is, constant) nerve firing from the various sensory mechanisms stimulated by gravity (semicircular canals, stretch receptors of calf muscles, etc). Without gravity there cannot be such constant stimulation. Even with exercises, this effect is only periodic. Also, stimulation to the postural fibers needs to be performed at a low level of activity, not at the higher levels of strength often used in exercises.

The teacher guides the pupil into positions of mechanical advantage to encourage the muscles to lengthen.

The Lost Sixth Sense

David Garlick makes a distinction between the five senses that are concerned with the external environment and the sixth sense, which conveys signals from the muscular system. Garlick argues that these signals from the muscles can be suppressed or "gated out" before reaching consciousness, and that the more we are preoccupied with the external world, the more likely we will be to shut out information from our internal world. Natural mechanisms, such as strong emotions, strongly contracted muscle, and the distracting influence of the external world, tend to "gate out" the sixth sense. These mechanisms excite the five senses at the expense of proprioceptive information. Furthermore, our body posture and movement programs do not require continued attention, so it is common to disregard the resulting sensory feedback.

With the Alexander Technique, red muscle fibers that have changed through misuse and overuse into white fibers are gradually converted back into red fibers. This means that the appropriate balance of red and white fibers in the body is re-established through lessons in the Alexander Technique.

Sensory Appreciation is the sixth sense that allows us to evaluate our limb and body position and movement.

HEARING

SIGHT

SMELL

TOUCH

TASTE

SENSORY
APPRECIATION

BREATHING

For any organism to function it needs energy. The chemical reaction that turns the food we eat into energy requires oxygen and produces carbon dioxide as a waste product. Oxygen is obtained from the air by means of the lungs. They are enclosed in the thorax, have a spongy texture, and can be expanded and compressed by movements of the thorax in such a way that air is inhaled and exhaled. As the lungs are thus ventilated, gaseous exchange of oxygen and carbon dioxide occurs between the air and the blood vessels in the lungs.

The average lung capacity of an adult is about 10 pints (5 liters), but in normal tidal breathing the exchange is only about a quarter of that. During exercise more energy and more oxygen are required so the capacity is increased. The thorax can never collapse completely, so there are about 3 pints (1.5 liters) of air that can never be exhaled. This is called the residual air. It exchanges carbon dioxide and oxygen by diffusion with the tidal air that comes into the lungs.

Inspiration

To inhale, the space in the thorax must be increased, causing the lungs to expand and draw in air through the nose and trachea. This is achieved by the diaphragm, the sheet of tissue separating the thorax from the abdomen. When relaxed, it is domed slightly upward. When the diaphragm is contracted, it flattens out, thereby increasing the volume of the thorax. The short intercostal muscles run from one rib to the next in a diagonal direction, away and down from the spine. When contracted they pull the rib cage upward and outward, thereby increasing the volume of the thorax.

Expiration

The lungs are essentially elastic, and once the thoracic volume is decreased, they will shrink back to their relaxed size, forcing air out again. To achieve this the diaphragm and intercostal muscles relax, allowing the diaphragm to return to its domed shape and the ribs to move downward and inward.

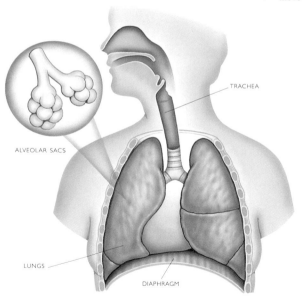

ALVEOLAR SACS

TRACHEA

LUNGS

DIAPHRAGM

Thousands of air tubes make up the lungs. The trachea branches into the bronchi, which divide into smaller tubes called bronchioles. These subdivide into microscopic alveolar sacs.

VITAL CAPACITY is the largest volume of air that can be moved in and out during ventilation.

RESIDUAL VOLUME is the air that remains after a forceful expiration.

VITAL CAPACITY

RESIDUAL CAPACITY

HOW THE VOICE WORKS

The vocal mechanism (voice) consists of three parts that need to work in coordination. A correct functioning of the primary control is the vital ingredient in making sure that the voice works efficiently.

1. The Energizer

The voice needs breath to work. It is like the wind in the sails of a boat, or the steady air underneath a bird's wings, providing the necessary energy for the boat to move forward and the bird to fly. *(See the section on "Breathing," page 54.)* Without breath there can be no voice. The efficient working of the energizer is dependent on the whole psychophysical mechanism.

The Physics of Breathing

BOYLE'S LAW

If gas is kept at a constant temperature, the pressure and volume are in inverse proportion or have a constant product. If air is confined at atmospheric pressure in an airtight container, there will be equal amounts of pressure acting on the outer and inner walls of the container and the differential pressure will be zero. Decreasing the volume of the container will increase the pressure inside with respect to the outside, whereas an increase in the volume of the container will decrease the pressure in the container with respect to the outside. In man, the lungs lie enclosed in the container of the airtight chest cavity (thoracic cavity) and communicate with the outside through the windpipe (trachea) and mouth (oral cavity). The structure of the chest cavity is such that its volume can be made to increase or decrease. Increase in volume of the chest cavity creates negative pressure in the lungs with respect to the outside (inspiration). Consequently, air will rush into the lungs until the inside and outside pressures are equalized. Decrease in the size (volume) of the chest cavity causes air to rush out of the lungs in the same way (expiration).

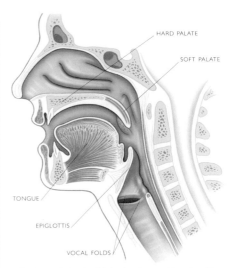

The larynx (voice box) is in the pharynx (throat) and is composed of several pieces of cartilage (Adam's apple). The trachea (windpipe) extends from the larynx to the bronchi in the chest cavity.

Posture, structure, emotion, and the situation you are in all play vital parts in how well the energizer functions.

2. The Vocalizer

Within the larynx, the vocal folds move together to make sound. This is facilitated by the muscles that attach to the laryngeal cartilage in such a way that they become more tense or relaxed. When they are tense, the voice is high-pitched; when they are relaxed, its pitch is lower.

3. The Resonators

Resonance depends on three conditions: the size of the space, or cavity; the number of openings off the cavity, and the actual structure of the walls of the cavity. The walls of a space correspond to the walls of a room. Sound is quite different in an empty room to one filled with furniture or people. Different materials affect resonance. Heavy drapes, cork insulation, bare wooden floors, thick carpets, all create different sounds. The inside of your nose (sinus cavity), mouth, and pharynx all affect sound differently. The spaces in your face, head, throat, and upper chest are all used as resonating chambers – they are called the pharyngeal, oral, facial, and nasal cavities.

THE PROCEDURES
THINKING IN ACTIVITY

MARCUS AURELIUS SAID that we become like our habitual thoughts. In the following procedures we are going to look at how you can begin to change your way of doing things. This is possible because you can employ the two principles of the Alexander Technique: inhibition and direction. Because you are unique, you will bring your own special talents and problems to every action you perform. Perhaps you will be quick to agree mentally with the principles explained in an idea, but slow to make your thoughts connect with your movements. You may be able to feel things in your body immediately, but not know how to respond to this feedback. You may be able to see the movement in your "mind's eye," but will not be able to manage the graceful rendition of your private picture.
There are a few lucky ones who will be able to think about, then see, hear, and feel the movement working together. This ability is commonly described as being talented, coordinated, skilled, or just plain lucky. Most of us need some help to achieve this state.

PRACTICE MAKES PERFECT
The Alexander Technique can help us achieve grace, poise, and full creative expression of ourselves.

Lessons in the Alexander Technique will help you to acquire the experience you need to get the most out of these procedures. It will teach you how to co-ordinate yourself more efficiently, save your energy, and boost your enthusiasm.

The ideal condition would be, I admit,
That man should be right by instinct;
But since we are all too likely to go astray
The reasonable thing is to learn from those
who can teach.
SOPHOCLES: ANTIGONE

Alexander teachers are trained to help you realize your responsibility for yourself. They guide you in the performance of everyday movements until you learn how to apply inhibition and direction for yourself. They are capable of noticing when you have reverted to your old habits. Habits are hard to break, but you can, with the help of a teacher, change the way you perform everyday actions. By using your own good sense, you can begin to think about "how" you use yourself. Bringing your conscious mind to bear on any action is not going to make you lose your spontaneity. By breaking your habitual patterns and reactions, you can make things easier for yourself.

God guard me from the thoughts men think
In the mind alone
He that sings a lasting song
Thinks in a marrow bone.
WILLIAM BUTLER YEATS: PRAYER FOR OLD AGE

The Movements

BREATHING

STANDING

Practice everyday movements using the Alexander Technique.

SITTING

WALKING

We have therefore to see that while carrying out these procedures we do not allow improper movements resulting from our bad habits to occur. Sherrington states, "Breathing, standing, walking, sitting, although innate, along with our growth, are apt, as movements, to suffer from defects in our ways of doing them," Alexander originally advised practicing, "before a looking glass in which to watch ourselves trying it." We can check bad habits by observation. Alternatively, a skilled instructor maintains the head in a proper, or less twisted, position relative to the neck, while the pupil consciously inhibits habitual movements (e.g. bringing the legs toward each other while sitting down or getting up) that interfere with its proper performance.

As you go through these procedures, try to be aware of your balance and poise throughout each movement. By breaking up the procedures into steps, you will be giving yourself a chance to consider the different positions that you adopt throughout the movement. As Professor Dart has said in *Skill and Poise*, "The movement of an acrobat or gymnast is performed by a body which at every phase of the movement i.e. the initial, intermediate and terminal positions is in a state of mobile equipoise or balance."

HEAD BALANCED FREELY

RIBS MOVING FREELY

The help of an Alexander Teacher is invaluable when first learning the principles of Conscious Inhibition and Conscious Direction.

STANDING

When you come up to standing, you need to think the directions that encourage the body to reach its full height and width. Allow the neck to be free so the head can go forward, and up so the spine can lengthen and the back can widen.

Because the lower limbs are used as weight bearers for the upper body, we tend to fix them into a rigid position and lock our knees to hold us up. Instead of using the legs as struts, think of keeping your neck free and your head going forward and up and your back lengthening and widening. This takes the pressure off the legs so it is not necessary to brace the ankles, knees, or hips. Now let your weight go down through your heels, but don't push back on your heels. Dropping your weight releases your lower back, and your hips are free to drop back and down. Avoid squeezing your toes, bracing your knees, or stiffening your ankles. The arch of your foot should be lively. The Chinese acupuncture point of the arch is called the "Bubbling Spring." The three weight-bearing points of the foot are the heel, and the points just behind the big toe and behind the small toe forming a tripod, the arch being the top of the tripod.

These are all preventive directions – they refer to what the body is naturally inclined to do when we stop interfering with it. Through these procedures and with the guidance of an Alexander Technique Teacher, you can refine your ability to register interference. You are not trying to correct your posture, but rather discovering how a dynamic posture emerges out of your awareness of what you do not need to do.

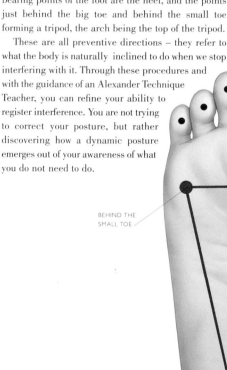

F.M. Alexander standing in his study in London.

BEHIND THE SMALL TOE

BEHIND THE BIG TOE

HEEL

THE TRIPOD DESIGN OF THE FOOT The weight-bearing points of the foot include the five pads of the toe for balance.

Standing

STEP 1

Have your weight evenly distributed between both feet. Allow your neck to be free so that your head can nod forward and go up while your back lengthens and widens.

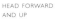

HEAD FORWARD
AND UP

STEP 2

Lift one foot off the ground and balance on the other foot. Experience the weight moving between the three points. Do not be frightened by feeling unbalanced. Repeat with the other foot.

WEIGHT EVENLY
DISTRIBUTED

BACK
LENGTHENS AND
WIDENS

WEIGHT TRANSMITTED
THROUGH TRIPOD
POINTS

KNEES FREE TO
GO FORWARD

STEP 3

Experience the weight moving between the two tripods. Now that you are back on two feet, remember the instability that you experienced when balanced on one foot. Experience the lightness and upthrust. Do not brace your knees.

WAY OF WALKING

*To take a step is an affair, not of this
or that limb solely, but of the total
neuro-muscular activity of the moment,
not least of the head and neck.*

CHARLES SHERRINGTON, 1946
THE ENDEAVOUR OF JEAN FERNEL

PUSH
OFF
POINT

TRIPOD

Being able to walk in the upright position is one of the great human achievements in the long course of evolution. When walking, it is important that you maintain the poise of the body by not collapsing down into your hip joints and stiffening your legs. Walking has a natural rhythm peculiar to each of us. We often recognize someone coming toward us long before we can see their faces by their way of walking. When we are feeling well or have something to look forward to, we walk with a spring in our step, gracefully and easily. Perhaps the opposite is seen more often. When we are ill or depressed, we become like Shakespeare's schoolboy "creeping like snail, unwillingly to school." The fact that we can move in the upright posture requires a balancing act. Our fear of falling is inherent within this subtle relationship between gravity and uprightness. This fear can tend to make us overcompensate by using too much muscular effort.

We need to become more aware of our feet and the part they play in the way we walk. As we walk, the arches of our feet act as shock absorbers. As the weight transfers onto the foot, we make the footprint. Then the flexors of the toes contract and the back foot is actively propelled forward. We usually walk on firm, even ground, with our feet protected by shoes. Therefore there is little need for our arches to adapt to different terrain. When we begin to expose our feet to more sensations, we keep the muscles active, which increases feedback. The study of Reflexology works on the principle that the feet represent the microcosm of the body, with all organs, glands, and other body parts laid out in a similar arrangement on the feet.

*Here comes the lady O so light a foot
Will ne'er wear out the everlasting flint*

WILLIAM SHAKESPEARE: *ROMEO AND JULIET*

"Walking on Eggshells"

Your feet play a very important part in how you walk. Think of what it feels like to walk on thick carpet or soft grass, or about walking barefoot on a rough wooden floor with possible splinters. Think of walking on rough terrain, uphill, down-hill, over stones. Did you tighten your toes to avoid stubbing them on the rough bits? Think about walking on the beach with burning hot sand. Did you spring onto the wet sand at the water's edge? Think of walking on icy pavements and in high-heeled shoes.

Walking only requires a small part of your available muscle power, so there is a reserve for you to use when some special action is required, such as walking upstairs, running, climbing a mountain. It is not necessary to make undue effort to walk if you are prepared to move. You need to look out and see where you want to go. The eyes lead the head and then the body moves.

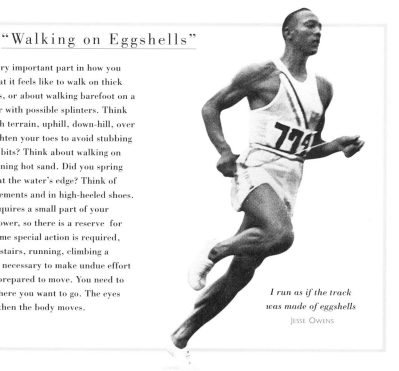

*I run as if the track
was made of eggshells*

JESSE OWENS

"The readiness is all"

WILLIAM SHAKESPEARE: *HAMLET*

DO

- Free the neck and let the head go forward and up.
- Free the ankle joints.
- Breathe out on the movement.
- Let the knees go forward easily.

DON'T

- Stiffen the neck.
- Hold the breath.
- Take a big step.
- Let your weight sink into your hips.
- Let your weight roll from side to side (rolling gait).
- Flatten the arch of the foot.

EYES LEADING
THE HEAD

NECK FREE, BACK
LENGTHENING

Walking

STEP 1

Stand equally with both feet. Breathe out and bend the knee forward. Lift up one heel, then put it back down again in the same place. Think of your spine lengthening up to your head and down to your feet. Repeat this movement with both feet in an easy rhythm on the same spot.

STEP 2

Let your heel come off the floor, and place your foot in front. Keep the weight still on your back foot with your front foot only slightly ahead. Be careful not to make too big a movement here.

STEP 3

Let your head move over your front foot and transfer your weight forward. This makes the footprint. Let the rear knee bend and the heel leave the floor. Do not move from side to side. Walk forward with an easy, flowing rhythm.

STEP 4

Do not stiffen your arms. Let them hang freely by your sides, swinging slightly in opposing directions to your feet. Left arm goes with the right foot, right arm goes with the left foot. The swing of your arms can make walking easier.

Walking Up Stairs

STEP 1
Stand with your weight equally distributed. Stop and breathe out. Bend your knee and ankle, raise your leg, and place your foot on the step. Think of going up, but leave the weight of your body wholly on your rear foot.

"Oh snail
Climb Mount Fuji
But slowly Slowly"
ISSA

Walking Backward

Try a new experience of walking. Look behind you and check that there is room to take a few steps. Step backward. Then place the next foot behind you and take another step. If you are having problems with your walking, taking a few steps backward can break the habits that may have been causing the problems. Rock back before stepping forward to remind you to stay back and not get ahead of yourself.

STEP 2
Let your head nod forward and up and lead your body diagonally up so your weight is transferred onto the foot of the first step. As this happens, your rear foot comes onto its toe and pushes off the ground.

CARRYING A LOAD

Suitcases seem to get heavier and heavier as we carry them. We try to release the tension in our arms by shaking them. We try to stretch out our backs by arching backward or forward as our muscles tire. We feel we need to apply even more effort. A vicious circle is set up. Before you lift, check you have not tightened your muscles too much.

BENDING

There are many ways of bending, and some are positively harmful. In every medical center there are leaflets giving instructions for lifting. The problem with giving the instruction "bend your knees so that you do not strain your back" is that when you simply bend your knees, your legs can take too much of the strain. Although the large muscles of the thighs are capable of taking a great deal of weight, they should not be overused when bending. It is important to consider whether the way you are moving is mechanically efficient. The definition of a good machine is "one that uses minimum effort to achieve maximum efficiency." When bending, you

Undue tension from carrying

want to reduce strain and subsequent wear and tear on the muscles, joints, and bones. If you involve your back muscles and your hip, knee, and ankle joints, you will be exercising your body and giving all your muscles a good stretch. As the muscles pull against each other, tone and suppleness are maintained. As your muscles lengthen, the habits of contracting and shortening are reduced. This increased efficiency can lead to less discomfort and pain.

DO

- Breathe out.
- Keep the thought of lengthening your muscles.
- Let the arms hang freely from your shoulders.

DON'T

- Tighten your neck.
- Have your feet too close together.
- Think of going down.
- Set yourself into a position.
- Stiffen the ankles and knees.
- Tighten in the front muscles.

Lifting

STEP 1	STEP 2	STEP 3
Free your neck and let your head go forward and up. Bend your knees and lower yourself with your arms hanging freely in front of you. Do not hold your breath.	Take hold of the handle of the suitcase. Do not grip it too tightly. Lift it a little way off the ground and check its weight. Put it back on the ground and breathe out. When holding the weight, allow your hips to go well back and your long back muscles to stretch.	Come to the standing position, bringing the suitcase with you. Be aware of maintaining your full length and try not to let your body weight be pulled over to the side of the suitcase. Begin walking in a measured rhythm.

Bending

STEP 1
Stand with your feet slightly
wider apart than for standing
(see Standing Procedure). Say
"No" to getting ready to bend,
and release your neck muscles so
your head nods gently forward.
Breathe out.

STEP 2
As your head nods forward,
let your knees bend and your
ankles bend. Your buttocks
move back and down in the
opposite direction by gentle
lengthening and stretching of
your back muscles.

STEP 3
Check your knees are pointing
away from each other. When you
have considered your knees going
forward and away, check again
that you have not stiffened your
neck muscles.

STEP 4
Allow your arms to hang freely
from your shoulders so your
hands are in front of your body.
Do not fix into a static position,
but keep the overall releasing of
your muscles.

STEP 5
As your muscles lengthen and
release, your ribs begin to move
in and out, giving more space in
the thoracic cavity and your
breathing naturally deepens.
Now say a whispered "Ah."

STEP 6
When you want to stand up,
say "No." Free your neck and
then go up until you are in the
upright position. Be aware of
how this way of bending has
increased your muscular tone
and suppleness.

SITTING

The ability to sit in the upright position is one of the most important developments in human evolution. For manual skills to develop, humans had to be in a stable position with their hands free. Most of the tool-making and tool-using activities of humans and of the great apes are carried out in the sitting position.

When seated, our bodies find more stability than when standing. Often we tend to sit badly, putting too much weight on our hip joints and internal organs and creating excessive pressure on the joints and disks of our spines and on our thighs. When we sit down to relax, it feels very comfortable at first. Taking the weight off our feet is a relief. However, as we sit, we often sag down. The longer we continue to sit in a collapsed way, the more likely we are to cause stiffness and rigidity. We have all experienced having to get up quickly to answer the door or telephone and finding that we are almost too stiff to move. We get pins and needles in our legs and feet. The reason for this is that we have moved from a collapsed, deadening posture to an active moving one and our muscles could not respond. We can avoid this by making sitting a more conscious process and not putting so much weight down onto our joints.

FREDERICK MATTHIAS ALEXANDER AND CHILD SITTING

Sitting

STEP 1

Use a chair with a level seat and put your feet flat on the floor. If your chair is too low, put something on the seat. If it is too high, put something under your feet.

STEP 2

Stand in front of the chair with your feet apart and your weight evenly distributed between them. Do not stiffen your ankle joints and knees. Let your head pivot forward from the top joint and breathe out.

STEP 3

Do not think of going down into the chair, but be aware of the two-way stretch of your back muscles. Let the hinge mechanism of your hips work in order to bring your head back over the spine so that you are seated in the upright position.

DO

- Sit on your seat/sitting bones.
- Release your ankles.
- Release your knees.
- Think of lengthening along your spine.
- Sit lightly.
- Sit with equal weight on each buttock.

DON'T

- Pull your head back.
- Stiffen your neck.
- Think of going down to sit.
- Hold your breath.
- Arch your back.
- Brace your legs to get up.
- Lower yourself with your arms.
- Pull down to get up.
- Collapse in front.

Ancient Egyptians knew how to sit.

Sitting in all types of chairs

A straight-backed chair with a flat, hard seat gives you clear feedback on your sitting position. The procedure for sitting in a soft chair is the same as for a straight-backed chair, but because the chair is soft, there is a lack of feedback. When we sit in soft chairs, we habitually switch off and end up in a crumpled heap. Relaxing need not mean collapsing. Put something behind your back if the seat is very deep and use the arms of the chair or sofa to keep you more upright. If you can put your feet up, so much the better.

By taking time to think how you sit, you can avoid postural problems.

STEP 4

There are two bony projections of the pelvis called the seat bones (ischia). They are a little higher than the lower edge of your buttocks. You should be sitting on them if your pelvis is in balance.

STEP 5

Your weight should be equally divided between the front of your foot and your heel. Your feet and calves should be vertical to your knees. Do not hold yourself up rigidly as the seat of the chair is supporting your weight.

STEP 6

Make sure your feet are flat on the floor and your ankles are not stiff. Let your head lead the movement by gently nodding forward so that your body follows your head and moves up in space.

READING

The earliest books were large and heavy. People needed to use stands with sloping surfaces (lecterns), on which to rest the books. This also allowed the books to be viewed at an angle that made reading easier on the eyes. The lectern is not essential for modern books, which are not as large or heavy, but having the book at an angle to your eyes is beneficial. It allows you to see

more efficiently and prevents the strain that can develop in both your neck and shoulders from looking directly downward. Resting the book on the back of a chair is a good way of improvising a lectern. When you are reading in bed, prop yourself up with pillows and bend your knees to form a natural slope on which to place your book.

A lectern provides a good angle for your book.

FREDERICK MATTHIAS ALEXANDER READING

Reading

STEP 1
Sit comfortably on the chair with your feet flat on the ground. Breathe out.

STEP 2
Do not hold yourself up rigidly, but allow the back of the chair to support your back.

STEP 3
Pick up the book and rest it on your knees with your hand keeping it open and breathe out.

DO

- Sit on your seat/sitting bones.
- Release your ankles.
- Release your knees.
- Think of lengthening along your spine.
- Sit lightly.
- Sit with equal weight on each buttock.

DON'T

- Pull your head back.
- Stiffen your neck.
- Think of going down to sit.
- Hold your breath.
- Arch your back.
- Brace your legs to get up.
- Lower yourself with your arms.
- Pull down to get up.
- Collapse in front.

Resting a book on the back of a chair is a good way of improvising a lectern.

When you are sitting on a soft chair, sit well back and put pillows behind you.

STEP 4
Lift the book by supporting the back of it with the other hand and hold it at an angle of about 45 degrees.

STEP 5
Try not to hold your breath (even when the story gets exciting).

STEP 6
Remember to put the book down on your lap and look up from the text now and then as this can stop you from overfocusing and prevent eyestrain.

HANDWRITING

Medieval manuscripts took time to write, giving pleasure both to the scribes and to those who read them. Pride was taken in having a good hand, and people were paid to write beautifully. Italic writing was taught in schools, but today handwriting is not taught as carefully. Many of us type our thoughts and miss out on the link between forming the letters manually and the satisfaction that a well-written page gives.

Today we write with a variety of implements – pencils, fountain pens, fiber-tipped pens, and crayons. One of the claims that a manufacturer makes of his pen is that it writes easily. We need to consider how we use the pen in order for this to be the case. Too often we create undue effort by holding the pen too tightly. It is helpful to practice picking up the pen easily and making some preliminary movements in the air before you put it to the paper to write.

A sloping writing surface creates a better angle for your eyes and helps to prevent you from collapsing down in front, putting undue pressure on your internal organs and breathing.

DO
• Have a good desk height.
• Have a sloping surface.
• Take time.
• Get up at regular intervals.
• Have equipment properly set up.
• Keep awake.

DON'T
• Collapse forward and hunch over.
• Hold your breath.
• Stiffen your wrists.
• Narrow your shoulders.
• Tighten your forearms.
• Go too fast.
• Grip your pen.
• Remain seated too long.
• Go into trance.

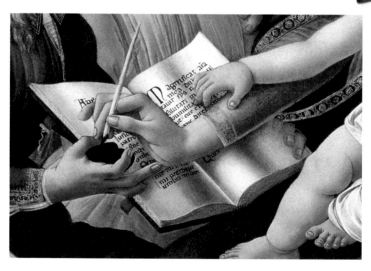

The sloping writing surface is important because the extra support helps to reduce tension in the forearm and wrist.

EXTENSION
Place the pen gently between the thumb and index finger.

FLEXION
Bend the thumb and index finger, moving the pencil up and down.

Handwriting

STEP 1
Check the height of the table or desk you are going to use. You need to be able to move forward freely from the hinge joints of your hips. Point your fingers down to the ground, then take hold of the chair.

STEP 2
Allow your head to nod forward and let your body move forward from the hinge joints of your hips. As you do this, slide your chair up closer to your desk. Breathe out and bend your arm freely at the elbow joint.

STEP 3
Allow the muscles to flex until you can place your hand on the table. Rest there for a moment, then slowly rotate your hand from the palm-down position (prone) to the palm-up position (supine). Keep your wrist free as you do this.

Italic Writing

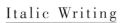

Italic writing requires the position of the pen to vary, which means that the pressure on the pen must change. Because the letters are not joined up, the writer has the chance to stop as he goes along. The pen has to be dipped in ink very often, providing more time for the muscles of the hand to recover from the fixed position of holding the pen. Writing was originally done on a sloped surface with the writer standing up.

STEP 4
Turn your hand over and flex it back from your wrist, keeping your hand straight so your fingers point directly upward.

STEP 5
Keeping them straight, flex your fingers forward from the knuckles. Now rotate your thumb around so it meets the pad of your index finger. This movement is known as opposition. Gently bend and straighten your finger and thumb. Repeat this movement a few times until it feels smooth and easy.

STEP 6
Place your pen by a simple movement between your index finger and thumb. Gently hold it, take care not to grasp it. Repeat the bending and straightening of your fingers and thumb with the pen in your hand. Put the pen to paper, take your time, and make some definite strokes.

USING A KEYBOARD

Although old-style typewriters, with their heavy action, have been replaced by better keyboards, using our fingers freely on a keyboard still presents many difficulties. Although we no longer need great muscular effort to push down the keys, typing still causes neck aches, headaches, frozen shoulders, and frustration. One of the problems we face when typing is the need to look at the document. Often as we peer at the paper, we cause stiffness by tightening the neck muscles. When audio-typing, we are tempted to go at breakneck speed. If we give ourselves a second for the sound to register before we try to type a word, we may have more success. We tend to hold our breath as we try to hear what is being said. As we work at a computer screen, we tend to lose concentration and go into a trance. Becoming aware of our breathing pattern can reduce neck strain in these difficult situations. As the flow of air keeps the intrathoracic cavities open, more oxygen can get to our brains. This not only helps to keep us awake, but enables us to be more conscious of what we are doing. Mindless activities often cause boredom. When we are bored, we make mistakes. Taking short breaks, even standing up for a moment behind your chair, can help.

MEETING A DEADLINE CAN CAUSE STIFFNESS AND TENSION

Using a Keyboard

STEP 1
Keep maintaining the two-way stretch of your back muscles. When your buttocks reach the seat, let the hinge mechanism of your hips work in order to bring your head back over the spine, so that you are seated in the upright position in the chair.

STEP 2
Stretch your fingers down toward the ground and breathe out.

ERGONOMICS

The design of the work space may be given serious consideration, but the design and function of the people using the work space is often ignored.

STIFF NECK AND
SHOULDERS

HOLDING BREATH

STIFF IN ELBOWS
AND WRISTS

RESTRICTING
THE BREATH

ROUNDED
SHOULDERS

COLLAPSED
IN FRONT

STEP 3

Breathe out and bend your arms freely at the elbow joints. Allow the muscles to flex until you can place your hands on the table, keeping your arms at right angles to the table. Rest there for a moment.

STEP 4

Begin as you did for writing, but this time, after flexing your hands back from your wrists, place them gently on the keyboard. When your fingers are over the keys you wish to press, say "No" to the thought of hurrying, free your neck, breathe out. Do not make undue effort and especially try not to tighten your wrists.

SQUATTING

Squatting is the natural way to raise and lower ourselves. Small children employ this way of getting up and down all the time, although later in life many of us lose the ability. Squatting is the simplest natural way to get close to the ground. If we did not have chairs to sit on, we would squat.

Squatting can be beneficial by giving a good stretch to the long muscles of the back and stimulating the soft internal organs (viscera) of the body. Many may feel that it is an impossible movement, but this is only through lack of use. As the general tone of your body improves and as your ankles become freer, then squatting does become possible.

CHILD SQUATTING

When a child squats, the heels are in contact with the ground. When our ankles get stiffer, we may find it difficult to keep the heels flat. If you can do this, you will create a good antagonistic stretch of the muscles.

Squatting

STEP 1

Stand with your feet slightly wider apart than for the standing procedure (see Standing, page 58). This helps to maintain your balance when you lower yourself to the ground. Say "No" to the feeling that you will not be able to squat.

STEP 2

Continue with these directions until you encounter any resistance in your muscles. Stop where you are and wait for a second, then see if you can continue. If you find further movement is not possible, stop where you are.

STEP 3

In the squatting position, allow your arms to hang freely between your knees ready for use (see Gardening, page 156; see Lifting, page 75). Stay like this for as long as you feel comfortable in order to give your muscles a chance to release into the new position.

STEP 4

When you decide to get up, think of where your head will go. It needs to move in a diagonal direction up over your feet. Do not overtighten your leg muscles.

LIFTING AN OBJECT (INANIMATE)

Do you remember going to the circus and watching the clowns struggling to lift the heavy dumbbells? Their unsuccessful attempts to move the weights were very funny. Then suddenly they were hitting each other over the head with the dumbbells, and you realized that what you had thought were huge heavy balls were actually made of foam rubber, painted to look like gray metal. When we imagine things are going to be heavy, we will find them more difficult to lift if we get ready with too much muscular tension. When we expect things to be heavy, we get ready with what we consider to be the appropriate amount of muscle tension.

When you grasp an object, the shape of your hand needs to change. The position that the hand naturally assumes to grasp an object is called the position of function of the hand. When the muscles and joints of the hand are in a state of equilibrium, promoting muscular efficiency, then we can grasp an object with

minimal effort. There are two things that can help you get into a proper position before you try to lift something. First, remember inhibition, and say "No" and remember to give your directions. Second, try not to expect the task to be difficult or impossible, then the lifting procedure can become a little easier if you move freely. Your body weight can become an effective counter-balance. By stiffening and fixing our muscles, we are often defeating ourselves before we begin.

Don't make undue effort... it is not as heavy as you think.

Lifting an Inanimate Object

STEP 1

Before you lift, pause for a moment and ask yourself whether you are generating unnecessary effort in preparing to lift.

STEP 2

Being careful not to grip too tightly, take hold of the object. When you grasp an object, the handle follows the life line of the hand. Bend your knees and lower yourself and take hold of the object. Lift it a little way off the ground and check the weight of it.

STEP 3

You may find that the move was easier than you had expected. By not stiffening your arms you have, not interfered with your breathing.

LIFTING AN OBJECT (ANIMATE)

When we have to lift a baby or a child, so often we hold our breath. Because we are frightened we might lose our grip, we tend to hold on too tightly. Our hands must change shape, but not to the extent that they become claws and by their excessive tension frighten the baby. We need to balance the weight of our body against the moving weight of the living object we are trying to lift. Because we feel we need to hold the baby close to us, we often create too much tension in our arms and shoulders. We can hold someone freely yet securely without tightening. Support and a feeling of security are given to the child through the feelings in our body.

SHOULDERS RELAXED

In order to lift a child safely, it is important to remain relaxed; otherwise, the tension in our bodies will be communicated to the child.

KEEP BREATHING

FINGERS MAINTAINING SHAPE

Lifting an Animate Object

STEP 1
Before you lift, pause for a moment and ask yourself whether you are generating unnecessary effort in preparing to do so. Pay attention to your neck and let your head go forward and up.

STEP 2
Being careful not to grip too tightly, take hold of the object. Lift it a little way off the ground and register the weight of it. When holding the weight close to your body, allow your hips to go well back and your long back muscles to stretch.

STEP 3
You may find that the move was much easier than you had expected. By not stiffening your arms, you have not interfered with your breathing or pulled down in front causing pressure on your internal organs.

REACHING UP WITH THE ARMS

We need to be able to reach up with our arms without incurring pain or even injury. We can strain our shoulders, and stiffness can result if we use our arms wrongly. If this misuse is persistent, "frozen shoulder" can be the result. The design of the shoulder is so flexible that problems in the joints and muscles are very common. The medial end of the clavicle, or collar-bone, is the only fixed joint for the whole of the arm and the only bony connection. The clavicle runs the width of the shoulders and of the upper body, and is at the center of movement of the arms.

The muscles provide support for the arms and allow for the movement of the hand (manipulation). When operating to raise the arm, these muscles can easily overtighten, and inflammation or tendonitis can result. This painful condition can make raising the arms even a small degree almost impossible *(see Tendonitis, page 46)*. If you need to get something out of a cupboard, use your eyes to look up without pulling your head back. You can look up without shortening your back and neck.

Ah, Man's reach must exceed his grasp,
else what's a heaven for?
ROBERT BROWNING

Reaching Up

STEP 1
Rotate your arms so your palms are facing forward. This anatomical position helps your shoulder girdle to release.

STEP 2
Turn your hand around so your palm is facing backward. Your shoulder girdle should move freely with your arm as an extension of your head, neck, and back.

STEP 3
Look up and begin to lift the arm by allowing your pointing finger to lead the movement. Try not to sway.

STEP 4
Raise the other arm so both arms are reaching up. Be careful not to lift your shoulders, and do not brace your knees, arch your back, or hold your breath.

STEP 5
When you have to hold a weight up with your arms, use your own body weight as a counterbalance and do not stiffen up.

DO

• Free the neck.
• Breathe out.
• Drop the shoulders.
• Lengthen the fingers.

DON'T

• Lift the shoulders.
• Hold the breath.
• Brace the knees.
• Overextend the elbow joint.
• Drop the head back.

LYING DOWN (SEMI-SUPINE)

Lying down is one of the quickest and simplest ways of allowing our bodies to come back into shape. This procedure has beneficial effects. It allows the spine to de-rotate and lengthen, and brings the head into a more forward position relative to the neck. In the supine position with knees bent, the pelvis can tilt backward and the lumbar curve flattens out. The spinal and abdominal muscles can release undue tensions, allowing gravity to have a beneficial effect on the diaphragm *(see Breathing, page 54)* and the ribcage to work more efficiently. A deeper breathing pattern happens, and the whole system calms down.

Without the fear of falling, the inherent elasticity of the body has a chance to reassert itself. If you lie down for ten to fifteen minutes each day, it will make an appreciable difference.

Lying Down

STEP 1

Put a book or some other support under your head. This needs to be about 2 inches/5cm high on the floor. Sit on the floor in front of the book or other support and breathe out.

STEP 2

Allow your spine to roll down onto the floor until the back of your head is on the book. Be careful that your neck is free and your head is not jammed against the book. Too few books will reduce the natural curve of the neck, and too many could push your chin onto your chest and restrict breathing.

STEP 3

Bend your knees and bring your feet near to your buttocks. You need to have your knees bent but not strained, so your lower back is not arched but is in contact with the floor. Place your hands on your lower ribs, just above your waist.

BACK IN CONTACT WITH FLOOR

KNEES BENT

FEET FLAT ON FLOOR

HEAD SUPPORTED

Benefits

- Releases muscles and joints.
- Takes pressure off spine.
- Releases diaphragm giving more rib movement.
- Allows for more regular breathing.
- Gives digestive release.

- Frees neck muscles.
- Takes pressure off eyes.
- Jaw releases.
- Unclenches the hands.
- Gives time to think and become more conscious.

STEP 4

As you lie in this semi-supine position, allow your whole back to be in contact with the floor. Be aware of the nine weight-bearing parts of the back – the head, the shoulders, the elbows, the hips (pelvic crests), and the feet. If you stop tightening your muscles unnecessarily, the ribs move more freely to allow the air to come in and out.

STEP 5

After about ten minutes, you will often find that your breathing has changed. When you begin to think about getting up, remember to take your time. Slowly raise one arm above your body so your fingers are pointing directly upward and then look to one side.

STEP 6

Let your arm lead your body so that you roll over onto your side. Stop and breathe out and check that you have not stiffened your neck or begun to overcontract your stomach muscles.

STEP 7

Move onto your hands. Rock forward and backward, allowing your head to lead your body forward. Say "No" to the idea of standing up. Bring one foot forward and put it in front of you. Allow your head to nod forward and your weight to move forward from the hips until you begin to move diagonally upward until you are standing.

CRAWLING

Crawling is one of the important stages in our development. Returning to being on all fours allows the head to move in the same direction as the spine, as is the case with animals. When an animal wants to move forward, the head leads and the body follows. If the back sags down, you will not be able to move forward easily. In order for the movement to happen, you have to allow your back to rise up. Some babies, who move from creeping to bottom bouncing, omitting the crawling stage, can have problems with reading skills later on (see *The Procedures of Professor Dart, page 88*).

Crawling is one of the important stages in our development.

Crawling

STEP 1

Stand with your feet placed underneath your hips. Take a small step backward. Bend your knees and lower yourself down onto your knees. Breathe out and check that you have not stiffened your neck at the end.

STEP 2

Look sideways at one of your hands by allowing your head to turn gently to the side, then move the hand and opposite knee forward. Do not lift either off the ground. Breathe out and allow your spine to lengthen and widen.

STEP 3

Look at your other hand, and then move your hand and knee forward together.

DO	DON'T

- Keep your eyes looking downward.
- Remember to rotate your head sideways before moving.
- Let your feet trail behind you.

- Arch the back.

- Let the back sag down.

STEP 4

Repeat left/right (cross-pattern) until a steady rhythm is established. Be aware of the diagonal connection through the back muscles from the left shoulder to the right hip and from the right shoulder to the left hip.

STEP 5

Stop moving and free your neck, then gently rock back onto your heels. Take your hands off the ground and sit back on your heels.

STEP 6

Let your head nod forward and come up onto your knees so you are in the kneeling position. Bring one knee forward and put the foot on the ground. Gently rock back onto your back leg and give a gentle push with the top of the foot.

STEP 7

Return to standing and be aware of the diagonal cross-pattern reflex.

MAKING SOUNDS

*"There is a kind of voice that accords with the ear
not so much by its volume but by its quality."*

QUINTILIAN VI (III)

The Alexander Technique grew out of the problem that Frederick Matthias Alexander had when he tried to make sounds. As a result of formulating his Technique, he found a new way to use his voice. One of the procedures which enabled him to do this was the Whispered "Ah." All voice teachers and singing teachers, including Alexander, have always valued the sound "Ah" as a measure of the effectiveness of the voice. The old singing masters understood that the ability to vocalize "Ah" was an important aspect of correctly vocalizing the other vowels. In order to produce a vowel you need a constant unbroken stream of air. Consonants, on the other hand, interrupt this stream of air and momentarily stop the sound by using the lips, tongue, and teeth to block the air. If you can speak or sing a good open "Ah," then the other vowels can become more open and free.

Whispering occurs when the vocal folds do not close along their entire length. Normally, we use our voices for speaking and are much less familiar with the whispered tone. Problems can be covered up by the spoken tone, and underlying problems in vocal functioning can be revealed when "Ah" is said in a whisper. Choosing to whisper the vowel "Ah" gives you the chance to break your usual habits of vocalizing. Combining "Ah" with whispering was an inspired procedure developed by Alexander. This procedure, which allows you control of the outbreath by whispering "Ah," is one that will repay daily practice. It can increase your length of breath and strengthen your voice. In addition to these vocal benefits, the exercise can calm you down, leading to being less anxious.

THE TIBETAN AH SYMBOL

Important parts of this procedure are the instructions to think of something funny that makes you want to smile or laugh. This has the physiological effect of lifting the soft palate, livening the facial muscles, and giving a message to the diaphragm to release. As tension in the jaw and face release, the pressure on the saliva glands is loosened, causing them to secrete saliva. This helps to prevent your mouth from drying out.

Putting the tongue against the back of your lower teeth is a preventive measure to help you stop retracting the back of the tongue and constricting the throat. It also creates a good antagonistic pull in that strong muscle. The tongue is the only muscle in the whole body connected directly to a bone (hyoid bone) and exhibits a persistent tendency to overtighten and retract, not only restricting the air flow, but creating a closed vocal tone that sounds strained.

The voice wheel is a way of visualizing the smooth flow of air necessary to good vocal tone.

Public Speaking

Do you feel nervous when asked to speak in public? Most people do. The thought can cause you to hold your breath, tighten your diaphragm, and gasp for air. You rush into what you have to say, to get it over and done with. By going too quickly, you do not give the vocal mechanism a chance to warm up. If you do this, it will be like trying to start your car on a cold morning – coughs and splutters – and no guarantee of getting out of the garage. The simple procedure of whispering "Ah" a few times before you speak helps with this problem. You will notice that at the end of your breath (Step 6) it is suggested you close your mouth and let the air come in through your nose. This stops any tendency at the end of your breath to gasp in air through your mouth. When you gasp, the larynx moves downward and is said to be depressed and your voice sounds strained. Because you are taking cold, often dirty and dry air straight into the mouth

ANSWERING THE PHONE
Take your time and practice the whispered "Ah" before you begin to speak.

You need a technique to deal with the unusual pressures of public speaking, at a wedding for example.

and throat, the vocal cords can become inflamed. To prevent this, the nose is designed as a very good filter system, which also warms and moistens the incoming air, so it makes much more sense to breathe through the nose. In ordinary speech and in performance, it is possible to allow the air to return through the nose while the mouth remains open *(see Breathing, page 54)* because of the oral seal. However, in this exercise it is useful to close the mouth after each exhalation so the inhalation is only through the nose. This re-establishes the nose as the most efficient and effective organ for breathing.

Try to do some whispered "Ah's" every day. Just before brushing your teeth could become a regular time to practice. You have the advantage of checking in your mirror that you have maintained your full stature and are not stiffening and pulling down. Another good time is when the telephone rings. This can come as a surprise, and you may react by stiffening and holding your breath. Instead of answering immediately, take a second and do a whispered "Ah." Because you have given your voice a chance to warm up, you will sound better.

TOOTHBRUSH DRILL
Take time each day to practice the whispered "Ah" in front of a mirror.

The Whispered "Ah"

STEP 1

Blow the air out through your mouth.
Do not stiffen your neck or tighten and pull
down as you exhale. Allow the air to return
through your nose. Repeat.

STEP 2

Think of something funny that makes you want
to smile or laugh. This is a very important part
of this procedure and needs to be practiced.
It is a simple instruction, but sometimes
people do not have the ability.

STEP 4

Put the tip of your tongue against the back of your
lower teeth. This is a preventive measure to help
you stop retracting the back of the tongue and
constricting the throat.

STEP 5

Open your mouth by allowing the jaw to drop
forward and down. Do not let the weight
of your head drop back and down. Say "Ah"
in a whisper.

STEP 3
Give your directions to free your neck and let the head go forward and up. The movement of the ribcage should be sufficient to generate widening in the whole torso. Do not tighten the abdominal muscles or pull down in the upper chest.

STEP 6
When you have come to the end of your breath, close your mouth and allow the air to come back in through your nose. As soon as the air has returned, repeat the procedure.

Tuning the Voice

1. Free your neck.
2. Let your head go forward and up.
3. Let your back lengthen and widen.
4. Think of something funny that makes you smile.
5. Put the tip of your tongue to the back of your lower teeth.
6. Let your jaw open.
7. Say "Ah" in a whisper to the end of a comfortable breath.
8. Close your mouth.
9. Allow the air to come in through your nose.

MASSITER MUSCLES

If you overtighten the muscles of the face, it makes it more difficult to allow the jaw to drop open.

Do three or four of these in a sequence, carefully considering each point as you go along. As you practice, you will find that each stage leads into the next one easily and that there is a continuous circular movement to the exercise. Doing some whispered "Ah's" will have a good effect on your voice, your breathing, and your general well-being. Performers find that whispered "Ah's" have a calming effect on them if they have been experiencing performance anxiety or stage fright. By doing whispered "Ah's," you give yourself time to think before you speak. If you have trouble sleeping, this simple exercise often has very beneficial results.

The thought of something funny naturally causes the smile.

The Star – Expansion Through Expiration

The voice cannot function to optimum capacity when the body is contracted. Taking and maintaining your full height allows the voice to work fully, preventing a strangled sound. The star exercise encourages you to fill your full space and experience your full vocal tone.

STEP 1
Stand with your feet hip-width apart and allow your head to nod forward and up. Rotate your arms so your hands face forward.

STEP 2
Think of your fingers drawing your right arm up until it is at a 45° angle. Let your shoulder release down. Think of your weight going down through your left leg.

STEP 3
Bring your arm down as you extend your fingers into the space beyond you.

STEP 4
Repeat step 2 - left arm - right leg.

STEP 5
Bring arm down.

Natural Support

The star procedure can lead to a greater appreciation of the diagonal pulls of the musculature that create a two-way stretch in the body. By practicing vocal exercises in the star position, you can begin to experience how important it is to release and lengthen through the body in order to engage the supporting musculature. The muscles of the abdomen need to work harder when you engage your voice with more energy. If too much effort is required of the abdominal muscles, the body is pulled down and the voice is blocked; if too little effort is made, there will not be enough energy to motivate the voice. Lengthening and widening helps the postural muscles to create a two-way stretch in the body. A two-way stretch in the body, active enough to counteract the effort in the abdomen, helps it to contract appropriately.

STEP 1
As you direct the weight of the body down through your feet, direct the fingers of your hands toward the ground. Rotate your arms so your hands face forward.

STEP 2
As you direct your fingers into the space beyond your reach, raise your arms to the horizontal. Release your shoulders as you reach with your fingers into the space beyond you.

STEP 3
Breathe out on the blowing sound. Close your mouth and let the air return through your nose. Repeat three times. Bring your arms down.

STEP 4
Raise your arms. Say "Ah" in a whisper. Repeat three times. Bring your arms down. Hum "mmm" falling from a higher pitch to a lower one. Allow the air in through your nose. Now hum "mmm" again, this time raising from a lower pitch to a higher one. Allow the air in through your nose. Repeat three times. Bring your arms down.

STEP 5
Raise your arms into the star position. Vocalize "Ah," falling from a higher pitch to a lower one. Allow the air in through your nose. Vocalize "Ah," rising from a lower pitch to a higher one. Close your mouth and allow the air in through your nose. Repeat three times. Bring your arms down.

THE PROCEDURES
OF PROFESSOR DART
PARALLELS BETWEEN ALEXANDER AND DART

BOTH MEN CAME from pioneering stock in Australia. They had natural curiosity and persistence, a talent for asking unusual questions and endeavoring to answer them, and a personal necd (Dart had a disabled son) which meant they had to find some practical way to help themselves. They both decided on the path of re-education: rather than learning something new, they were rediscovering something forgotten.

PROFESSOR RAYMOND DART

had extensive knowledge of Man's progression to upright posture. He later wrote "Perhaps the richest comedy presented by the evolutionary process is that creatures nature designed to have perfect posture and vision should today represent a picture of bespectacled decrepitude."

By starting on the floor, he began to explore movement with no fear of falling. He made notes daily as he localized creaks and aches and other sensations, and became more aware of weight-bearing body parts. He warned that some people who try this out may see the movements as "ludicrous because they are infantile."

When he was living and working in South Africa, Dart, along with his two children, had lessons in the Alexander Technique. His son suffered spasms, and Dart dearly wished for his coordination and quality of life to improve. As an anthropologist, Dart already

Lying on your back, side, or front gives enormous sensory input through the skin, stimulating our sensory "map" of ourselves. Touching surfaces can become pleasurable, as this "wakes up" the sensory nervous system.

The hairline of the head contacts the ground. The arms fold at the elbow crossing the chest.

The torso rests on the folded legs and the ankles cross each other under the tail.

Pause when the body is poised ready to fall and note any tendency to hold the breath. Exhale with a whispered "Ah."

When rolling over, move as slowly as possible. Notice the difference when the eyes are open or when they are closed.

The first two vertebrae (atlas and axis) are built to allow both nodding movements of the skull on the atlas...

Twisting action can only occur by differentiated action between flexor and extensor action in several body segments.

...and rotational (left and right swinging movements) of the skull and atlas upon the axis.

Use Both Sides

While experimenting with these movements, Dart heard cracks or other audible noises as muscles let go of the joints they had been jealously guarding. Dart describes this as the:

capacity of the synovial fluid to form gas bubbles, and the subsequent physical modifications in the quality and surface tension of the synovial fluid, enables joints, which for years have moved little if at all, to assume gradually, or even rapidly, the mobility they were fashioned to experience.

When crawling, by exploring moving one limb at a time, first one side, then the other in a slow progression, we notice that when we want to move faster, our opposite limbs move in a cross-pattern fashion. Dart observed: "I continually discover my own faulty techniques to lie in passing too rapidly over basic essentials and rushing ahead to performance of stardom."

From crawling we can explore the transition backward and upward, one leg extended out to the side, so we can arrive at a sitting position, balancing on our seat bones. As babies this is our first experience of being upright unaided. We can explore both variations to left and right with the opposite legs extended and flexed, one rotation

seeming easier for us than the other. This is because we have a dominant side related to our preferred hand, and, if overindulged, over the years we begin to develop twists. We have two interwoven spiral sheets of trunk musculature directly attached to the skull: when both spirals are working in a balanced way, there is general lengthening and widening; when not, there will be scoliosis. Dart always advocated using both sides of the body and both sides of the brain, so as not to become too habituated to using only our preferred and therefore biased side.

When in a semi-supine position we can explore movements of arms and hands by resting the backs of the arms and hands on the floor, and stroking the backs of the hands on the floor, moving from the wrist and then extending this flippering action to a movement of the whole limb from the shoulder, or the lower arm from the elbow. We can then roll onto our side, looking for a spot to place our farther hand, and then bring ourselves up and over onto our hands and knees again. From this quadruped position, we can explore being on five weight-bearing points in a form of Muslim prayer.

With this extra head contact, we can release any unnecessary tightening in our armpits and thus open up our shoulders – "Relaxation of the unwanted muscles is the key to skilled performance."

CASE STUDY

JEAN CLARK
Alexander Technique
Training Consultant

Over the years I have gained a better sense of my bones and joints and a realization that the muscles that clothe my skeleton have over an extended period of unconscious misuse become a too-small suit of clothing, reducing my flexibility and full range of movement of my joints. One of my early movement excursions was crawling (also called creeping) on my hands and knees. From this experience of being a quadruped, I began to see more clearly Alexander's insistence on the importance of the head, for now mine truly was out in front taking the rest of my body with it, and if I did not overtighten my neck, my spine had a chance to lengthen out in the direction of my forward movement. It highlighted, as I could see if I looked sideways into a mirror, that I had become used to tightening in the middle of my back, so that on all fours it dipped down (as in the poor Marx Brothers' horse, but less drastically), but if I could really promote my Alexander directions, my back could lengthen and widen, rather like a table top, and my knees moving forward and away also helped my lower back to become better sprung. Occasionally, on my crawling expeditions around the house, I would meet my surprised cat on his own level,

seeing the world from his point of view. For me it was a limited view, and I could see afresh how as babies we wanted to see more. Dart has said that early humans developed upright posture because they wanted to extend their range of vision. I recaptured this urge to see more and could explore the transition of using the new found power in my back to bring me back and up onto my feet. Tucking the toes under facilitates the movement, and the backward and upward progression can be continued in my thoughts even when I am up to my full height. This helps me offset the tendency in general living to pull myself forward and down. Coming upright gives me more range of vision and greater range of movement, but as most of my interests are going to be centered in front of me, I must continually renew my backward and upward direction that maintains my lengthening spine and freely poised head, so I do not squash down onto my vertebral disks, interfering with my shock-absorbers, nor reduce the space in my joints. I have found also that, with improved physical balance, I can better overcome psychophysical (or psychosomatic) fears and gain a measure of evenness of mind and temper – equanimity.

Mankind can only look ahead
as far as he can look back.
RAYMOND DART

Weight-Bearing Points

SEMI-SUPINE. The back of the head is supported by books. The hands are resting on the lower abdomen with elbows pointing away from each other. The feet are placed about hip-width apart.

PENTIPEDAL. The forehead, elbows, and knees are on the floor. The center of the forehead is in contact with the ground.

CROUCH. The hairline of the head contacts the ground. The fingers wrap around the base of the neck.

CREEPING. The weight of the body is supported by the hands underneath the shoulders and the knees under the hips.

Let's see how they move...

PART THREE

Constructive Conscious Control

EDUCATION

PERFORMANCE SKILLS

SPORT AND RECREATION

Everything that has these...

also has these

They are spirals and they are everywhere

They are powerful

CONSTRUCTIVE
CONSCIOUS CONTROL
EDUCATION

To come into possession of intelligence is the sole human title to freedom. The spontaneity of childhood is a delightful and precious thing, but in its original naïve form it is bound to disappear. Emotions become sophisticated unless they become enlightened, and the manifestation of sophisticated emotion is in no sense genuine self-expression. True spontaneity is henceforth not a birth right, but the last term, the consummated conquest of an art – the art of conscious control, to the mastery of which Mr. Alexander's book so convincingly invites us.

JOHN DEWEY, INTRODUCTION TO *MAN'S SUPREME INHERITANCE*

The Alexander Technique is based on the belief that we could do more to help ourselves. It is a means of re-educating ourselves so we can learn more easily, and retain and use what we learn. Education is a continuing process of asking questions.

"How do we work?"

"Could I be more productive?"

"Am I using my time and myself well?"

In these ways we can begin to explore our potential. The journey from being in the womb, through birth, babyhood, childhood, work, family life, and old age can, we believe, be helped by the Alexander Technique.

Give a child conscious control and you give him poise, the essential starting point for education. Without that poise, which is a result aimed at by neither the old nor the new methods of education, he will always be cramped and distorted by his environment. For although you may choose the environment of a nursery or a school, there are few indeed who can choose their desired environment in the world at large. But give the child poise and the reasoned control of his physical being, and you fit him for any and every mode of life; he will have wonderful powers of adapting himself to every and any environment that may surround him.

Knowledge is experience; everything else is simply information.
ALBERT EINSTEIN

Everything that makes our language unique [and us human] flowed from the simple capacity to impose a delay between a signal, a message, or an event that we experience and our reaction or response to it.
JACOB BRONOWSKI

PREGNANCY and BIRTH
ILANA MACHOVER

Pregnancy brings with it far-reaching changes in the woman's body and psyche, which affect body use and are in turn affected by it. Tension, back ache, and varicose veins are common complaints. The sooner a pregnant woman begins her Alexander Technique lessons, the better she will be able to cope with the changes and alleviate the complaints. The Technique can also make a crucial contribution to achieving natural childbirth.

Childbirth is a very finely tuned involuntary process. It is regulated by a series of signals exchanged between the mother's brain and the rest of her body. The contractions of the uterus are controlled by the secretion of the appropriate hormones during each of the three phases of labor: dilation of the cervix, birth, and afterbirth of the placenta. But this natural process can easily be disrupted (or halted all together) by inappropriate psychological, physical, and chemical inputs. For example, dramatic change in the laboring woman's environment, pressure of other people around her, or continuous monitoring can all cause anxiety – and anxiety releases wrong hormones.

Any end-gaining behavior in this process is self-defeating, since the mother cannot control directly her autonomous nervous system and her hormonal balance. During the first stage of labor the woman does not "do" anything: the dilation of the cervix happens by itself, and she only needs to allow the process to proceed. With each contraction, by moving in a relaxed way and agreeing to accept the pain, she can help herself to cope.

During labor it is very difficult for the unprepared woman to accept that the pain of the contractions is "normal." For the majority of women, this is the most severe pain they have ever experienced. Our society does not teach us to tolerate pain, and we are used to taking pain-killing drugs. However, these derail the natural process of birth by masking the body's signals and blocking their pathways; this often makes further medical intervention necessary, leading to forceps or caesarean deliveries. In order to accept labor pain as normal, we have to understand its role: labor pains are not pathological but functional.

This triumph is not to be won in sleep, in trance, in submission, in paralysis, or in anesthesia, but in a clear open-eyed reasoning, deliberate consciousness, and apprehension of the wonderful potentialities possessed by mankind, the transcendent inheritance of a conscious mind

F.M. ALEXANDER: MAN'S SUPREME INHERITANCE

Crawling Improves Coordination

Crawling as taught in an Alexander Technique lesson is very beneficial during pregnancy and is a good preparation for childbirth. It helps to calm you down and control minor aches and pains. A few minutes every day will make you feel great:

1. Start from kneeling on all fours.
2. Take one small step forward on diagonally opposite limbs, say right hand and left knee, then left hand and right knee.
3. With the head leading, crawl, and let your body's weight shift to the limbs that were in front, and are now stationary.
4. Crawl slowly and rhythmically.
5. After crawling, stay for a while on all fours and gently rock the body to and fro.

Conscious Control of Pain

In this the Alexander Technique can be of enormous help. Through inhibition and direction *(see Inhibition/Direction, page 14)* we can stop our habitual reaction to pain. Instead of flexing, tensing, and pulling our heads back and down (followed by other symptoms of panic attack), we can consciously and voluntarily undo the involuntary muscle tension. We can learn to exercise conscious control over our posture and movement, giving us an indirect conscious way of affecting the hormonal balance.

This is far from easy, since the startle reflex *(see Startle Pattern, page 179)* is so often activated. We acquire the habit of going into this startle mode whenever we are stimulated to movement. Consequently there is a lot of unnecessary muscle tension in most of us most of the time, especially during movement. It takes time to re-educate the body and replace habitual patterns of tension with those of release. But having learned to move in her daily life without interfering with the primary control, a woman in labor can apply this skill during contractions. There is no need to be athletic or to perform complicated positions or exercises. Most of

these only enhance patterns of tension and misuse and encourage an attitude of end-gaining *(see End-gaining, page 35)*.

We cannot expect a woman in labor to undo the harmful habits of a lifetime without previous careful preparation. When pregnant women have lessons in the Alexander Technique, they are preparing for Eutokia, which in classical Greek means a happy, relaxed childbirth. It is now widely accepted that a woman should move freely and stay upright during her labor. The dynamic posture of bending *(see Bending, page 64)* is one of the best stances during pregnancy and is particularly advantageous during labor. In this position, as the mother leans forward, her abdominal wall becomes a kind of hammock for the baby, while the tilt of her pelvis makes more space for the baby's head to enter the pelvic brim; thus the baby is encouraged to move into the optimal position for birth. At the same time, the force of gravity – the weight of the baby – aids contractions and makes them stronger and more efficient. To soothe the pain, it is of paramount importance to be able to move freely, so during labor this posture ought to be used in a dynamic way: the woman can maintain her primary control while shifting her weight from one leg to the other, either on her own or supported by her partner.

The dynamic posture of bending is one of the best stances during pregnancy.

The tilt of the pelvis is able to allow more space for the baby's head to enter the pelvic brim.

The Pear Movement

Ilana Machover, who runs classes in Eutokia, says: "Since many women find it helpful to go on all fours during labor, I looked for a way of making this stance more dynamic and integrating it with the principles of the Alexander Technique."

1. The woman is on all fours and with her head leading, her body describes the shape of a pear parallel to the floor. This shape echoes the outline of the uterus.

2. The pear movement is useful in encouraging her to free her joints and prevent tension from accumulating, especially in the shoulders, arms, and lower back.

3. With her neck free and her head leading the movement, her back lengthens and widens, so it does not sag and create tension in the lumbar area.

Salivation

Salivation is one of the means toward achieving a relaxed state of mind and body. The body of woman in labor gets a signal that a contraction is about to begin. At this moment she should first think of a smile and allow her mouth to become wet. Thinking of something funny produces a smile, releasing the tension in the jaws and face. This loosens the pressure on the salivary glands and causes them to secrete. This is a preventive measure, so the mouth does not become dry. Dryness of the mouth is a symptom of a panic attack. Here, the practice of the whispered "Ah" is very useful.

CASE STUDY

ANNE GIRLING
Student of Eutokia Birth Method

The Alexander Technique is all about being aware of how you move and therefore making the movements less wasteful of energy – vital during labor. Resting, which slowed down labor, worked, too – it was nice that these things really do work, and I could even appreciate it at the time. I rested on the floor, lying on my left side, the way I had been taught in the Eutokia classes. Getting off the floor to move during the contractions was imperative. I remember thinking how it was all in a good cause – each contraction was agony but bringing the baby. Ilana didn't say it, but I heard her voice in my head – I was fully lucid in between contractions to know this was a true and valuable thought to have, and the periods in between contractions were so clear and calm.

The Eutokia message is to avoid a rut and use all those movements that are helpful; to inhibit the urge to curl up and hold the breath, and instead to use the Alexander Technique directions. And to have someone remind you of them when you think you would rather forget them is wonderful! Practicing the variety of movements during pregnancy is very important so you have them ready in your mind. My memory is that I needed help to move out of a position that was slowing down labor into a more upright position (i.e. walking). I was resisting getting up toward the end of the first stage because I'd found a position on all fours – leaning on the big gym ball and banging it – that was helping me. I knew I should walk, but I didn't want to, because I was afraid to increase pain and speed up contractions. However, when Daniel did help me up and paced with me, it was refreshing both physically and psychologically.

Again, I don't remember ever feeling out of control, even when I was in second stage. When I could not resist the strong sensation of bearing down, I naturally went on all fours. My moans (whispered "Ah's") when I was "pushing" her out sounded good and actually calmed me down as I went through the contractions. Hannah was born about half an hour later – my beautiful baby.

GROWTH AND DEVELOPMENT OF THE CHILD

Prevention Is Better than Cure. We should try to give children the supportive atmosphere free from stress in which they would have time to learn about inhibition and direction and to practice these procedures. As babies they had "I want" as a basis for behavior. As they grew up, this was replaced by what their parents, teachers, or peer pressure wanted – how they should behave and what they should do led to a succession of don'ts. Negative commands imposed from the outside can break down a child's natural inhibition. The role of the Alexander teacher is essentially that of a facilitator. The ordinary stereotype of a teacher does not apply. Teaching becomes a learning situation in which both are students.

Learning is a process by which behavior is modified in the light of experience.

First Three Months

In the first three months of the baby's life, lack of head control is the important factor in how he moves. He develops the grasping reflex.

At Four Months

At approximately four months, he has head control – he takes pleasure in his own voice, he plays with his hands, he smiles at all faces. He sits upright unsupported with his hands free to play.

At Seven Months

At seven months he is sitting up with his back shaped in a single curve – he explores his environment with his eyes and begins to take solid food.

The Following Months

In the following months he becomes mobile, he crawls, he learns to come up from squatting to standing, at first holding onto things for support and then unsupported. He often stops halfway in the bending position. He comes up onto his toes. He stands, he walks, he explores, but always with his mother close at hand. He becomes quite a sophisticated problem solver by the end of the first year. All humans and animals show a tendency to walk in circles if they are blindfolded, as in the dark of night, in thick fog, or in a dense forest. Walking in a perfectly straight direction necessitates constant correction of deviation with the help of the eyes. The "circling instinct" is very noticeable in young children and young animals, and in the early stages of life it is no handicap because it always leads the infant back to his starting point whenever he becomes disoriented in his first exploration of the world. This instinct is most probably linked to the labyrinth of the inner ear, which provides an important part of the information that assists the balance and posture of the body. He experiences pain with teething. He learns to speak and recognize visual symbols. He moves away from his dependence on his mother; he starts to ask "what is that and why?" Children learn by copying. It is very important that parents and teachers provide good examples for children to copy. They need to be well coordinated and balanced and display ease of movement. When these things are happening, concentration is possible. If the people around them are disturbed or overtired and tense, children pick this up.

BALANCE AND EASE

Discipline and Structure

Do not let your eagerness to help deprive your child of finding out for himself. If you think of learning together, rather than you being the teacher and him being the only one who is learning, the whole process could be more fun. Children are eager to find out about everything, but they do need a calm atmosphere and a caring environment in which to learn. They don't respond to being told, but need to know. We need to find ways to arouse and keep their interest.

Children are very seldom bored. They do not mind how many times something is repeated. Each time it is new for them; each moment is different. They enjoy sensory stimulation. If we are happy to be in the moment and not thinking of doing something else, we will not be bored.

There is a growing trend to confuse virtual reality, that is, what we see on film, television, and computer games, with real life. If we passively watch children climbing a tree on a screen, it is not the same experience as climbing a tree. We miss out on sensing the feel of the bark, the movement of our limbs, looking where to put our foot next, the smell and sounds of being up in the leaves, even the real fear of falling. If we substitute television for real life, growth and development will suffer.

Parents are every child's first teachers. Long before children go to school, parents are guiding them through the early stages of the learning process into the extraordinary world of words, numbers, pictures, and the imagination. The Alexander Technique is concerned with the quality of learning and respects the fact that every individual learns differently. To open up the Alexander Technique to children and make them interested to learn, we have to start at the very beginning, and that is with teaching them inhibition or the ability to say "No" before performing even the simplest action. There is a game that is fun to play with children in order to re-establish "No" in a positive way. Ask a child, "Do you know the magic word?" "No," he replies. Children are delighted when you assure them "That's right, 'No' is the magic word. It can be your secret word. You can say it before you do anything. You can say it before you speak. Nobody needs to know that you are doing it. It is a secret that you share with yourself." This opens up for children a new way of thinking about the word

Our deepest learning comes from real experience, of the world outside, of Nature, and of others.

"No." For a child, the idea of inhibition and stopping needs to have a positive element about it. "No" usually means something negative. When children's understanding of "No" changes, they can begin to think about direction.

The Golden Thread

Most children have a fine sense of natural direction. Once they have stopped doing the wrong thing, very often the right thing does itself. For a child, the word "direction" could be described as a "golden thread running all the way from the top of your head to the soles of your feet, like a bright, shining ribbon, that you do not want to squash or crumple."

By preventing children from developing harmful habitual patterns that impede their health and progress during childhood, we could avoid some of the problems that then beset us as adults. We are often tempted to help our children to walk sooner than they are ready. Mechanical baby walkers are a bad idea since they can give the sensation of movement before the child has the necessary muscular development to cope. Folding strollers are equally inappropriate as the spine is collapsed and unsupported, thereby restricting the child's breathing mechanism.

Virtual reality is no substitute for the real thing.

TEACHING
THE TECHNIQUE
IN SCHOOLS
SUE MERRY

The characteristic note of true happiness is struck when the healthy child is busily engaged in something which interests it

F.M. ALEXANDER:
CONSTRUCTIVE CONSCIOUS CONTROL

Children start to alter their natural good use when they begin school. When you look at your child working and playing in school or at home, try to observe the whole child. If he is performing an intricate task with his hands, also look at what he is doing with the rest of his body. If your child is collapsed over a drawing or piece of written work, he cannot be coordinating well between hand and eye. If breathing is impaired, he cannot be functioning as well as he might. Feelings of low self-esteem, negativity, and of repeated failure can result.

Our education system is geared toward end-gaining. There are levels of assessment to be achieved, scores to go for, and examinations to be passed. Even kindergarten children are expected to be able to gain certain ends. So although you may be looking for your child to produce good-quality schoolwork, do you have the same interest in what he is doing with his whole

Fit the chair to the child, not the child to the chair.

self in order to produce such work? The pressure to master a skill and to produce work that gains approval can be a major contributing factor to deterioration of the use of the self. If you ask your child to try hard to write well, he will simply add more muscle tension to the activity. This is very unhealthy and can very quickly become part of a habitual way of writing and difficult to change. It produces not better, but more tortuous, handwriting.

Furniture

It is very noticeable how preschool children valiantly attempt to use themselves well – which is their natural use at this age – while attempting to cope with a chair that is far too big and badly designed to allow them to have good use. It is from this uncomfortable situation that we then ask them to perform.

When chairs are too big for children, they are forced to sit with their legs dangling uselessly. You can experience how uncomfortable this is by sitting on a high platform such as the kitchen counter. Sitting like this seems to put a certain amount of strain on the lower back. It is also a very unstable position. If you hold your arms out in front of your body, you will tend to tip forward. Imagine your child in this position with a desk before them. The arms will be used as a support for the

A collapsed posture restricts your breathing. When you are taking an examination, your brain needs all the oxygen it can get.

Wrong Formula

Try harder = do more = increase misuse
= intensify the conditions that are hampering
the achievement of a desired end
= be unhappy with the result = try harder =
give up = feel you have failed

WHAT IS A CHILD ACTUALLY LEARNING?
1. How much muscle tension in the whole body the activity requires.
2. How to relate to the desk before them.
3. The perspective to view the paper on the desk.
4. How to sit in the chair provided.

body and, as this puts quite a strain on the arms, it is easier to collapse forward onto the table so that the head and upper torso are often also supported by arms on the table. The feet and legs should be supporting the torso, and most very young children strive to get their feet onto the floor at first by sitting on the very edge of the chair. It is natural for most children to seek this connection to the floor through the feet. The natural way of sitting for most young children is in a squat with both feet beneath the torso and flat on the floor.

Children very soon become used to an unnatural way of using themselves when working at a table. They begin to learn bad habits. Such bad use is also habitually associated with whatever activity they undertake while sitting at a table. This is why when children grow and the chairs that they are using are the right size for them, they will usually still sit with their legs dangling uselessly, trailing on the floor, often wrapped around the chair legs. Consequently they will collapse down and use the table in front of them for support. For children to use themselves well while writing, they have to relearn how to write since writing, has become associated with bad use.

Classroom chairs seem to be primarily designed to stack neatly. Usually they are designed with a seat that slopes downward toward the back of the chair. This raises the knees higher than the hips and makes it even more difficult for the child to get his feet flat on the floor, The hips tend to slide to the back of the chair. As it is then very difficult to sit upright, the tendency is to lean against the backrest of the chair.

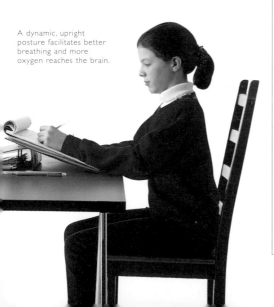

A dynamic, upright posture facilitates better breathing and more oxygen reaches the brain.

CASE STUDY

SUE MERRY
Alexander Technique Teacher,
Kingston Primary School

What I often see when a child sits working at a desk is that bad use becomes more difficult to change as time passes. I often see children with their feet not flat on the floor, often with their legs in all manner of contortions. Sometimes their torsos are slumped, and they are often leaning heavily on the table with their arms and even their heads. Their writing arms are usually very tight, probably because they are gripping the pencil. This is largely due to lack of awareness.

When working with nursery children we have a tremendous advantage because they are mostly still using themselves very well. All we really need to do is to draw this to their attention in a very positive way and make it possible for them to maintain this good use. The same work seems possible with older infants.

I have been working with these problems since 1994. It can be fairly easy through the Alexander Technique to reactivate this good use for them using images, games, stories, songs, and a small amount of hands-on work.

It is not an impossible task to teach a child that before he picks up a pencil or crayon, he simply stops first and checks that he is sitting in a tall way. The child has to understand the feeling of sitting in a tall way with the help of an Alexander teacher. This way every child could be learning a new skill with good use as an inseparable part of that skill. This does not mean not giving praise for good work, but to first give praise for good use. It is also a very beneficial experience for a child to be allowed the time and space to lie semi-supine for a very short time each day.

This approach to learning means changing the way that we think as parents, children, and teachers. It is probably much more difficult for adults to do this since we have so much more to relearn. It would mean trying to change yourself as much as your child. With the help of a qualified Alexander teacher and with the understanding and enthusiasm of teachers and parents, it could be possible in primary schools.

KEEPING LEARNING ALIVE

Teaching methods are based on the assumption that the student's conception of a new idea is identical to that of the teacher. Students frequently suffer disappointment and failure in their studies because they do not understand what is required of them. Every day in life misunderstandings occur in trivial as well as very important matters. This process of reasoning is inseparable from what we call "understanding" or "mental conception."

We expect students to acquire knowledge and to be put "right" in matters where they are judged to be "wrong." Parents have their own ideas regarding what the student needs now and in the future, and choose a school accordingly.

The student is asked to "sit up straight," "speak out," "take a deep breath," "see how quietly you can walk." These are specific end-gaining instructions that rarely include the means

Too many instructions can confuse the mind.

Wrong Way to Solve Problems

Exercise Teachers and parents mistakenly think that physical exercises, posture training, and breathing exercises will rid children of psychophysical defects. A student's harmful habits acquired during study cannot be remedied by physical exercises.

SPECIFIC CORRECTION Attempts to remedy a specific defect in a badly coordinated student, for instance, in handwriting, should take into account the standard of general psychophysical functioning in the student; otherwise, new faults will develop and old ones will be reinforced.

Sit up straight
Speak out
Take deep breaths
Walk quietly

whereby the student can carry them out, so they are made to feel it is almost a disgrace to be wrong. Teachers do not know how to prevent bad use in the student.

Overexcitement of the fear reflex has a very serious effect upon how the student is breathing, which is so closely linked up with the emotions. (As Byron wrote: "Breathless as we stand when feeling most"). These are tremendous impeding factors in the student's activities. In attempting to improve his handwriting, for instance, new faults will be developed in his general use, and established defects will become more pronounced. Knowledge acquired in this way is gained at the cost of losing coordinated control, particularly in breathing. The student then lacks the natural equipment essential to the best efforts to learn. The gradual lowering of breath during studies can result in a trancelike condition.

We cannot expect the best results in learning if the student's psychophysical functioning is inadequate. The student's early efforts to learn the curriculum are based on specifics, that is, on "end-gaining" principles of "trying to be right": long before adolescence is reached, this "end-gaining" procedure will have become established. There will be a reticence and resistant attitude toward accepting new ideas and experiences. There can be a serious deterioration in memory. These defects may account for the general lack in many adults to be able to learn and retain information.

Knowledge is of little use in itself; education gives us the ability to link up what we know with our new experiences. The ability to link up ideas is a measure of intelligence and is inseparable from the process of remembering. The value of knowledge lies in our power to associate it with the greater body of knowledge that should have come to us through our years of experience. We begin to substitute reason for instinct and reduce what Professor Dewey calls our "emotional gusts."

GROWTH AND DEVELOPMENT OF THE ADULT

The American philosopher and educationalist Professor John Dewey, who died in 1952 at the age of 92, was deeply impressed by the practical benefits and scientific soundness of Alexander's teaching. He said in *Use of the Self:*

CASE STUDY

MARY LUTYENS
Novelist and Biographer

Our family has a long connection with the Alexander Technique. First, my maternal uncle, Victor, Lord Lytton, knew Alexander well. He was a pupil of his and greatly admired him. Then my daughter benefited from the Technique for several years until she moved to the country, where the improved condition of her back enabled her to make the garden she longed for. My granddaughter, Anna Pallant, has been using the Technique in her work as a masseuse. It was Anna who introduced me to my Alexander Technique teacher, Glynn Macdonald. Let no one think that it is ever too late to learn. I was over 80 when Glynn took me on, and now at 89 I greatly look forward to my weekly lessons, to keep me mentally alive as well as physically supple. My mother and grandmother both lost their memories two years before they died. This is a fate I feel confident of avoiding with the help of the Alexander Technique.

Frederick Matthias Alexander at his 70th birthday party, with Victor, Second Earl of Lytton, Civil Lord of the Admiralty.

Education is the only sure method which mankind possesses for directing its own course. But we have been involved in a vicious circle. Without knowledge of what constitutes a truly normal healthy psychophysical life our professed education is likely to be mis-education.

Education continues throughout life. As we grow older we need not fall into the trap that, as we become less able to do as much as we could, we stop trying. Our life expectancy is much greater today, 75 years as compared with 47 years at the beginning of this century.

We can continue to learn new skills and apply the Alexander Technique to how we learn them. Our later years can be educationally enriched.

PERFORMANCE SKILLS
IN THE ARTS

What a piece of work is a man.
In form and moving how express and admirable.

WILLIAM SHAKESPEARE: *HAMLET*

The word "form" has two meanings. The verb "to form" means to mold by discipline, to train, or to instruct. The noun "form" means the shape, arrangement of parts, or the shape of the body. When the form of an athlete, musician, or even a horse is discussed, it is the state of health and condition of training that is being judged. They can be in good form, top form, on form. When we speak of people being in good spirits, we say they are in good form. The ancient Greeks made less distinction between the performing arts and the medical sciences. In Greek mythology, the children of Zeus were the muses who created music. Aesculapius was the inventor of medicine and Orpheus, with his lute, was the keeper of song and its healing powers.

Performers in the arts have always valued the Alexander Technique as a way of avoiding tension. In *Indirect Procedures*, Pedro de Alcantara said "The word tension has acquired an unwarranted, negative connotation. When somebody complains of tension, he really means too much tension, or more precisely, the wrong kind or amount of tension, in the wrong places for the wrong length of time. In itself, tension is not negative. 'Tension is a proper adjunct of human behavior – one cannot live without it,' wrote Patrick Macdonald. 'Tension creates and sustains life and carries it forward. Tension – of the .right kind – is a prerequisite of dynamic, energetic, vital human endeavor.'"

As you become less certain of the position you hold, you become more open and receptive to other possibilities. Artists often speak of having an inspirational experience. They felt they did nothing, but something came through them and they achieved a performance greater than they ever imagined they could; joyfully they were surprised.

Performance of any kind demands a high level of energy and coordination. In the mastery of their art, performing artists need directed body use and refined attention to achieve coordination. The Alexander Technique helps to develop a very high level of sensitivity and awareness in performers. Then they can begin to discover and discard unwanted postural, movement, and vocal habits that interfere with their art. Scientific research is confirming that efficiency of breathing, movement, and vocal coordination depend to a large extent on the ease and energy of the upright posture. Being unaware of this results in self-limitation, not just in physiological functioning, but in achieving full potential as a creative, intelligent human being. The Alexander Technique believes there is a connection between full physiological stature and full stature as a creative artist. The human instrument is the only instrument which cannot be tuned by someone else. We can get help from a teacher, but in the end we are the instrument, the player, the tuner, the artistic piece itself, and also the listener.

When once our grace
we have forgot,
nothing goes right.

St. Theresa of Avila

Full height, full width, full stature;
full readiness to act.

*Singing and acting, like the fine dexterity of a
juggler, with his cups and balls, require a shaping of
the organs towards a finer and finer certainty of
effect. Your muscles - your whole frame - must go like
a watch, true, true to a hare. That is the work of
springtime, before habits have been determined.*

GEORGE ELIOT; DANIEL DERONDA

In this section, the word "posture" will be used.
Posture can have the connotation of being static, not
dynamic. The term "dynamic posture" suggests a
readiness to act. Children, athletes, laborers,
artists, and dancers apply to their special
activities some phases of dynamic posture
they have discovered for themselves or been taught
by their instructors or coaches. Dynamic posture as
a part of posture generally, related to the everyday
activity of each of us, is new and has received
little or no attention. Good dynamic posture means
using your body in the simplest and most effective
way, using muscle contraction and relaxation,
balance, coordination, rhythm, and timing as well
as gravity. The smooth integration of these elements
of good dynamic posture results in neuro-
musculoskeletal performance that is easy, graceful,
satisfying, and effective.

Performance Strategy

PREPARATION ● ACTION ● RECOVERY

INHIBITION AND DIRECTION: Observe the
manner of preparation; accept that impulses
can be counterproductive; stop to establish
a readiness, an openness, a willingness
to communicate.

THE DESIRE TO PERFORM: Identify the
wish to perform, the character's need or
purpose; this will elevate your energy level,
increase lengthening and widening; breathe out.

ANTICIPATION: Think about the
performance; continue to give preventive
directions - "When I go, I will not disturb my
neck any more than necessary."

GO MEANS GO: Give up trying to get it right,
and allow things to happen, accept the
unknown, open to the unexpected.

RETURN TO STILLNESS: Inhibit and direct
to re-establish full stature; reflect on the
performance and ask the questions, "Did I
stiffen my neck and pull my head back any
more than I needed to?," "Did I end-gain, did
I do unnecessarily, did I force my responses,
or were they true to
the moment?"

Do not try
too hard. Return
to stillness and
allow things
to happen.

ACTING
PENNY CHERNS

An actor has to find a way of locating the differences between himself and the character he is playing. He needs to identify the kind of behavior and life choices the character makes and to discover how these are revealed in the interaction. One of the key tasks of the director is to enable the actor to absorb the character choices.

Preparing for a rehearsal is a vital area; it is necessary to let go of the outside world in order to focus on the task in hand. The Alexander Technique helps to find this new space and centers the actor so he can enter the spirit of the character. The actor's instrument is his body; an instrument has to be tuned so that any note played on it has a clarity and a resonance; the better the quality of the instrument, the richer the note. Language is like

TRAGEDY AND COMEDY

music; it has rhythm, energy, and a variety of sound patterns. Every individual uses language differently; the actor has to let it flow through him and his senses so it can resonate and reveal the text. The Technique helps actors to open themselves to this resonance.

When the actor is using his back, he is able to release the breath that gives vocal power as he experiences the moment. He will be neither ahead, behind nor beside himself, but can create from within himself.

Being within yourself also allows for spontaneity; this means that you are not responding on automatic pilot. You are free to respond to the interaction; the ability to receive and then change the energy is the very essence of being in a drama – like in a good ball game.

Blocking the other actor's input is like not listening in an argument, considering the alternatives, and having the courage to change your point of view. When improvising, this allows for spontaneity and giving the other actors a chance to contribute their ideas.

Having prepared, the actor can now be in the moment. For the actor there are, however, still hurdles to be crossed before the performance. The first is that moment in rehearsal when he knows his lines and the moves, but having discovered them, and that they work, he is tempted to fix the work. At this stage it is quite often possible to see the process that is evolving; a lot of energy and expression is going on in the facial musculature, but no real energy is flowing between the actors and everybody seems to be operating with the front of the body only. If the actor can be encouraged to let go and trust that the work has fully infiltrated himself, his performance becomes more free. The Alexander Technique allows the actor to be free and in the moment.

A production of *Bye Bye Birdie* at LAMDA in 1982. Courtesy of John Haynes.

CASE STUDY

PENNY CHERNS
The London Academy of Music and Dramatic Art

I am a theater and television director and acting teacher. I came to the Alexander Technique 15 years ago. When I started to have Alexander lessons, the changes in behavior became as apparent to me as the remarkable changes in my body and the improvement in my asthma. I began to change physically in such a way that I could not easily re-create my old physical habits and became increasingly aware of more subtle problems in my physical make-up; at the same time I became aware that I was able to prevent (later "inhibit") automatic responses to situations and have a moment of making a choice. It was this concept of making choices that I began to connect more fully to the acting process. I have always been keenly involved in this process, and have been considered an actors' and writers' director and latterly have developed work as an acting teacher. As a director I think it is important to drop the concept of "blocking" the play – a term used colloquially to describe how the actors are moved. The passivity of the image and its fixity are blocks in themselves. Helping the actors to place themselves, to find the dynamic energy of the piece and of their impulses is what the director is really doing. It is providing the tracks so it is safe to travel. I have progressively learned more about the acting process over the years because I have been increasingly open to understanding it through the connections I have made since I have been studying the Technique. It has not only been of enormous personal help, but it has informed my work. I believe it to be a key method of improving acting and performing and of immense use to actors in understanding the best ways of using themselves.

DANCING
PERI ASTON

*There is nothing constant in the universe – all ebb
and flow and every shape that's born bears in its
womb the seed of change.*

OVID: *METAMORPHOSES*

Without movement there is no life. Words applied
to the death state include "stiff," "rigid," "cold."
However fixed or blocked we appear, there are still
thousands of movements going on inside us – flowing,
pulsating, breathing, beating. When approaching
movement, our problems can be: stiffening, straining,
pushing, collapsing, pulling up, pushing down – this
blocks energy and stops fluency.

It is so hard to move fluently out of a fixed state – it
requires a huge amount of effort. We need to connect with
the inner flow which takes us easily into movement. The
outer movement is a continuation of the inner movement.

The root of the movement is the response to gravity,
giving grounded support. Like a tree, the roots form the
connections with the earth; the trunk gives flexibility

Movement is:

- an impulse
- a flow of energy – a space to feel the effect of
  gravity, the body's spring mechanism, a spiral
- a response to a stimulus requiring movement
  away from or toward expansion or contraction
- a moment of suspense
- falling in space
- responding to the contact of the ground

---

and stability, and the branches are like the arms
supported by the roots and trunk. There are three centers
of the body from whence you move – the gut, the heart,
and the head.

Consider the intention of your movement. When the
intention is clear, then the inner thoughts and feelings
are conveyed in the movement; there will be clarity,

glide revolve pull twist stroke cringe bounce flick sway glide
press thrust slap grind jerk slither

Movement is the essence of life
and vitality, encompassing many
different moods and desires.

connection, and communication. The moment of preparation to move comes from a still point. The Alexander Technique defines this moment as inhibition. This creates the possibility of choice:

1. to let go of any unnecessary stiffening
2. to think in which directions you want to go
3. to connect with the intention

When you do this, whatever movement you create will have a unity. There are so many qualities of movement. What unites them is "how" we prepare to move.

Making a quick, strong, pushing movement does not need to be tight, tense, with a lot of effort. It is still a movement of expansion from the center; the head is still freeing forward and upward and the feet letting go into the ground. Conscious control is continual inner exploration, paying attention to what is happening in this moment, not to what you think you want to happen in the next moment. By continuing to say "No," you allow yourself to expand, lengthen, and widen, and you leave yourself open to creative discovery.

Ask these questions as you move:

1. What do I intend by this movement?
2. What do I want to convey?
3. What moves me to move?
4. How does the body want to express it?
5. Where does it want to go?

CASE STUDY

PERI ASTON
Performance Artist and Alexander Technique Teacher

I always danced, but I was never quite a "dancer." The discipline of ballet was unreachable for me, and forced me into shapes that twisted and contorted my body as I tried harder and harder to get it right.

I was never quite a mime. I trained for three years in "mime" at Drama College, but it might more aptly have been called expressive movement. I came to contemporary mime technique late, after having children, and never managed to do the three-month/two-year intensive course. I just picked up bits and pieces along the way, struggling to get it right.

I was never quite an actress either. My confidence and voice were ruined at college by attempts to keep my ribs raised while breathing "on the diaphragm." I became afraid to speak.

I started my own creative work again 15 years after leaving college. But I still struggled with my body, pushing it to do things I thought it ought to do. I hung onto the old procedures – hard physical warm-ups, pliés, grands battements, the things I knew. I went on stage tense, and came off in pain, frightened by the clicks in my spine and the strain in my legs.

Then I began my Alexander training and slowly things started to change. First of all, my spine stopped clicking and fixing when I did that certain twisting movement. I prepared for performance by semi-supine and standing thinking. Altogether my body was fitter, more supple and flowing, more integrated. I have come full circle, I am dancing again. At age 55, I have become a dancer, but the kind of dancer I want to be, not what I think I ought to be.

As you from faults would pardoned be,
Let your indulgence set me free
WILLIAM SHAKESPEARE: THE TEMPEST

MUSIC AND MUSICIANS

For musicians to enjoy performance as much as the audience they require a well-practiced technique.

Musicians are people who have learned how to listen. Careless rapture does not mean that you do not care, but suggests music played with skill and joy. Creating music should not be stressful, causing you worry and making you overcareful. There is an old Chinese saying that the birds of worry and care fly above your head – this you cannot prevent; that they build nests in your hair – this you can stop.

Frank Pierce Jones, in his article on musicians entitled "Awareness, Freedom and Muscular Control" says:

> *There are musicians – some say there were more of them in the past – who get as much pleasure from a performance as they give, who always perform easily and well... There are others, however, with equal talent and training, to whom performance and even practice are exhausting, and whose professional lives are short because they lose the mastery of the skills they have acquired. They put forth more effort involving technical problems than the results warrant, and ultimately discover that they have used up their reserves of energy. If they understood the use of themselves as well as they understand the use of their instruments, such breakdowns would be far less frequent.*

Tuning the Orchestra

The orchestra is brought into accord by tuning each individual instrument. The quality of the whole relies on the sum of the parts being played by all. Harmony is achieved in this world of sound by increasing the players' awareness of the music, of themselves, of their instruments, of their colleagues, and of the conductor.

Flute
Watch that your head turns freely and do not shorten your neck. Breathe through the nose where possible.

Percussion
Watch your balance so you can move freely Use the weight of your arms to contact the instruments. Use the mallets as an extension of your arms' length.

Piano
See Piano, page 119.

Horn
Be careful about resting the instrument and pulling down in front.

Violins
See page 116

Viola
See page 114

Oboe
See page 121

Bassoon
Watch that the
instrument does not
pull you down.

Harp
Watch that you
keep your length
and width so that
your instrument
does not cause
you to lose your
balance. Keep
your legs and
lower back free
as you play.

Clarinet
Watch that you do not pull
down and hold the
instrument too firmly. Do
not overtighten your wrists
and thumbs when playing.

Trombone–Tuba
Watch that you do not lift
your shoulders and
shorten your neck. Do not
come down to breathe
and bring your instrument
with you.

The Royal Academy of
Music Symphony Orchestra

Conductor
Watch everything!

Cello
Watch that you maintain a good
contact with the chair and have a
long wide back. Do not grip your
instrument too tightly with your
legs, but let it balance freely.

Double Bass
Watch that you maintain
your full length and width
when standing or using a
stool. Keep your arms freely
moving from your back.

CASE STUDY

DOROTHEA MAGONET
Royal Academy of Music:
Learning the Alexander Technique
in Music Colleges

Young people enter music conservatories, colleges, and academies having undergone an intense period of practicing and auditioning to enroll. They then may spend many music lessons unlearning faulty playing or singing techniques they have acquired during the early stages of their music learning. The time music students spend practicing, rehearsing, auditioning, playing for competitions and performances increases dramatically. In addition to improving their music skills, they are also under pressure to attain high levels in academic studies.

During regular lessons in the Alexander Technique, students can discover how their habitual and ingrained ordinary thought processes influence and determine their physical use and how this can interfere with the acquisition of good technical skills and the desired expressiveness of their music. Under the guidance of a teacher, the student can explore means of stopping this vicious circle of unconscious and repeated attitudes, postures, and movements, which often are accompanied by excessive tensions, stresses, and tiredness, and thereby develop a new awareness that can lead to improved general use.

As the attention becomes more organized and action more coordinated, the student can respond appropriately to the perceived stimuli. This improves the music student's ability to learn and to take on board new instructions and information. Confidence and sensitivity increase, and greater clarity of thought may lead to more concordance between musical intention and technical accomplishment.

The principles of the Alexander Technique provide sound mental skills for the young musician to prevent unnecessary stress and injury; to improve stamina to deal with nervousness before and during performances; to enhance their ability to learn new music; and to make long rehearsals more interesting.

Many music schools, colleges, conservatories and academies offer lessons in the Alexander Technique either on an introductory basis or as a foundation course.

Conscious practice
refines mental
skills as well as
physical dexterity.

Learning how to Learn

The musician needs to understand how to use the instrument he plays. Too often attention is paid to tuning his instrument, while the equally important job of "tuning" himself is neglected. Another common mistake that the musician makes is that of diverting his attention from the playing itself so he tries to think of something else to "relax his nerves." Neither of these is satisfactory and often leads to physical discomfort and tiredness. Things are further complicated if he thinks the piece is difficult – all the old fear responses are generated, and he can end up suffering from pain that can often become debilitating as "nerves" that literally stop his playing. As he begins to employ the primary control, improvements enhance his ability to hold in his mind the complexity of the musical text, the overall shape of the piece, and the sounds he can create. The freedom and release in his back, neck, arms, and fingers provide the possibility of a true rendition of the notes. The miraculous coordination of body, mind, and spirit find their fulfillment in making music.

Anatomical Information

The two main masses of muscle, the extensors and flexors, need to be properly stretched out to create the antagonistic pull which maintains the upright structure. The muscles when operating with the opposing pulls create good tone. They are able to act and are ready to act, but do not actually need to do very much. The alternative is to have them both overacting and engaged in a real tug of war. This leads to "pulling down" and stiffness – not recommended for the musician who is trying to play in tune and get the fullest "tone" out of his instrument. When the muscles are overstretched, the musical tone will tend to be sharp. When the muscles are flaccid and understretched, the tone will tend to be flat.

Pitfalls of Playing

Try to avoid bracing the knees and overarching the back.

Try to avoid stiffening the neck, holding the breath, and having the feet too close together.

Try to stop collapsing in front and narrowing the shoulders

CASE STUDY

GRAHAM GRIFFITHS
Viola Player and
Alexander Teacher

Being a member of the busy Philharmonia Orchestra, I needed to find a way of playing the viola day after day with as little strain on my body as possible. I already practiced yoga and T'ai Chi, but I felt that by learning the Alexander Technique I would be able to use my body in a more economical way and be able to achieve the maximum result with the minimum of effort in my playing and in my everyday life. By not allowing a build-up of tension in the body, I hoped to avoid the physical problems suffered by most players at some stage in their careers.

After the first lesson I was sold on the Technique! I could not believe such changes could be made in such a subtle way. The release of tension gave me a sense of freedom I had not felt since childhood. Not only did I find practicing T'ai Chi much easier, but also, when I took my viola to the Alexander lessons, I found that I was making a more resonant sound. After a short time I enrolled at an Alexander school to train to become a teacher myself!

Gradually, playing in the orchestra became easier, and I was able to cope with the demands of conductors in a more detached way. I noticed that as my posture improved there seemed to be a knock-on effect upon the players around me.

In addition to being essential for me as a musician, the Technique has had far-reaching effects on many aspects of my life.

Good, released upright posture with open shoulders and appropriate stance leads to better playing.

An orchestra is only as good as its weakest player. Each member needs to consider and tune both his instrument and himself.

PLAYING STRINGED INSTRUMENTS
FELICITY LIPMAN

Felicity Lipman, who is Professor of Violin at the Guildhall School of Music and Drama, London, England, and founder of the Haydn Trio, believes that poise is the ability to move in any direction, at any moment, and at any speed.

Many people think it is necessary to "brace" themselves to stand. In fact, the more we allow our weight to release into the ground, the more the ground will support us and the easier it is to stand. The more we let the ground support us, the less we need to support ourselves.

When we stand with our arms by our sides, the weight is evenly distributed over the soles of the feet. When a violinist plays, his arms are forward and the weight needs to be distributed differently i.e. centered more toward the heels to counterbalance the arms. If this doesn't happen, the violinist will usually tilt the pelvis (we see an unnaturally hollowed back), thus completely altering the relationship of the head, neck, and back and spoiling the integrity of the spine. This restricts breathing and movement of the limbs, and prevents us from releasing body weight into the ground and from receiving the support of the ground.

It is common for a violinist to be unaware that he leans forward or cranes his neck forward or raises his left shoulder in order to reach the violin. These habits completely alter the relationship of the head, neck, and back, causing tension. If we can stand in a natural state of balance ready to receive the violin, then we can play with freedom and poise. We feel freer, lighter, when we allow the ground to support our weight. Poise in violin playing comes first of all from a redistribution of weight to accommodate the arms as well as our contact with the ground. This results in a flow of energy, eases the weight of our shoulders down the back and into the heels, and allows energy to rise up the front of the body. The concept of a dynamic flow of energy seems to help much more than merely demanding relaxed shoulders. This is an action rather than a posture.

Violin playing is a much more complex skill than that of standing! However, we can use the same supporting principles. There is a supportive opposition to our weight from the ground – we do not need to push our weight into the ground in order to stand. Similarly, the violin rests on the collarbone, and the head rests lightly on the chin-rest to prevent the violin from slipping sideways. The left hand cradles the neck of the violin. The relationship of each of these contacts is a dynamic one, as with the violinist's hand on the bow.

Many people think that the violin and bow are inanimate. In one sense they are, but seen from this perspective, just as in allowing the ground to support us we gain poise and freedom, so the very solidity of the violin and bow allows us this same poise and freedom to play music. The dynamic relationship of the bow's horsehair on the string is a most stimulating one. Each of these surfaces has an elastic quality. The horsehair bow has a natural springiness that varies along its length. The same can be said of the string (nearer to or further from the bridge). The subtle interplay of these two surfaces creates an ever-changing palette of colors. Our inner concept of music, together with our desire to communicate it, lets us explore this rich and varied palette.

RELEASED POSTURE ENCOURAGES FLOW OF ENERGY THROUGH THE BODY

The relationship between the ground, the performer, and the instrument is dynamic and fluid, a subtle interplay of energy.

GROUND SUPPORTS WEIGHT

CASE STUDY

FELICITY LIPMAN,
International Performer and Teacher;
Associate of the Royal Academy of Music;
Founder of the European Suzuki Association

I have experienced many eminent violinists over the years saying what was the "right" or "natural" way to play the violin. Unfortunately, there were major fundamental, physiological differences in understanding, and in the content of their teaching. Why should violinists have a detailed and practical knowledge of physiology? This is not their specialty. Many violinists based their whole teaching on what was appropriate for their individual body, ignoring the fact that there are many different body styles and each bow is unique. In 1992 I resolved to do my Alexander Technique training with Walter Carrington to gain not just a professional knowledge of physiology but a working knowledge – an experience of natural use of the body. Another of my reasons for training as an Alexander Technique teacher was the realization that I lived inside a body I had been taking for granted for decades. Like many musicians I was used to going for my goals with little or no attention to how my body was feeling – the musical idea or thought was paramount. This realization encouraged me to "inhabit" every nerve fiber in my body. During my training I became aware of tensions and imbalances throughout my body – notably in my neck, my shoulders, particularly the left, and in my pelvis and my legs. I gradually learned how to let go of unnecessary tension by studying

FELICITY LIPMAN

a means through which I could release them. I certainly learned all that I had hoped for in my Alexander Technique training – and more! For three years my body had experienced finding what "poise" is. I left the course with a desire to feel at ease and comfortable with any action. I have learned to be aware of tension and to understand the process of releasing it. I have a new sense of balance and of poise and a freer flow of energy. This has had a profound effect on my violin playing and teaching, which has become less authoritarian. After all, no teacher knows how a pupil's body feels. Teaching violin techniques, I tend to demonstrate the desired actions while the pupil watches not just the individual body part concerned, but how that fits into the whole pattern, e.g. if a child is staring fixedly at my fingers, I ask him to stand back and look at all of me and how the action of the fingers relates to the whole body; then I gently guide the child's limbs in the correct motion and finally ask him to "put it into the computer" i.e. make himself comfortable with the new actions. My teaching language has changed. I tend instinctively not to select words that could indicate forcing or tension but those which keep the whole body free, open, and energized with less about posture than about the feeling of the body in motion. The child absorbs dynamic posture as part of the flow of the movement.

The relationship of the hand to the instrument is essential for good playing.

PLAYING KEYBOARD INSTRUMENTS

To play in harmony with other musicians, you must try to find the harmony within yourself.

Understanding and using the instrument well are important considerations in being able to realize your musical skills. The tone of the muscles affects the musical tone that you are producing. A state of muscular harmony in which you are using the muscles in a coordinated way is necessary if you are going to be able to realize the harmonic potentials of the music. The dictionary defines harmony as "the agreeable effect of apt arrangement of parts."

Before you come to play on a keyboard, it helps if you understand some of its geographical detail. You see all these notes that look the same. In fact, they are all different and arranged in a pattern of white notes interspersed with black raised notes on a large flat area about four feet long.

The music from which you will play is placed above this keyboard. Instead of the score mirroring the keyboard, going from side to side, it is written from top to bottom going from up to down. In order to read the music, your brain has to involve itself in the sophisticated task of translating vertical instructions from your eyes into horizontal actions that you perform with your fingers and arms.

This takes a great deal of physical practice as you learn the sounds of low and high played on a flat surface.

To avoid undue stress, it is important that you familiarize yourself with the music before you attempt to play.

Reading music can often cause you undue anxiety. You tend to peer at the manuscript, narrowing your body and your eyes. This is the exact opposite to what is needed in playing. In order to cover the span of the notes, you need to widen through your back, shoulders, and arms, and feel in your fingers for the sound that you want. All the time you keep a regular pattern of breathing going. When you are faced with a difficult piece of music, one of the first questions to ask yourself is whether you have really understood what is being asked of you. What do these notes tell you about pitch; what do these patterns tell you about rhythm? You need to spend time analyzing and practicing the music in your head before you come to the practical task of playing the notes.

The mechanism of the piano is made up of keys that are mobile. In fact, if you just let your fingers touch the top of the keys, they make no sound at all. The key when touched has its own balanced movement to a certain place where it connects with the hammer that is going to contact the string. When you want to make a sound, you have to put pressure on the key to give it the necessary impetus for this contact. Different qualities of tone – soft, loud, velvet, ringing – need different sorts of pressure. Your mind's ear hears a certain sound which it would like to produce. Over time you begin to build up a repertoire of sensory appreciation in your eyes, ears, and fingers that allows you to become more skilled at this art of playing.

COLOR STAFF
MARGARET HUBICKI
PROFESSOR AND EXAMINER AT THE ROYAL ACADEMY OF MUSIC, LONDON

In the early sixties I invented Color Staff to help two very gifted eight-year-old string playing pupils of mine. One was a violinist who easily read the treble clef but not the bass, and the other a cellist who read the bass clef but not the treble. To help each of them share their knowledge of these clefs, I put together material for their fingers to feel, as well as their eyes to see the patterns forming the staff.

This material includes a board with five lines printed on it as well as one with two staves of five lines with a space for middle C. On these boards the different symbols of musical notation can be placed so that the learning of musical theory can be "played with the fingers" in a way that deepens an awareness of what is being studied. A board with the keyboard printed on it is also provided for clarifying and experimenting with the geographical pattern of black and white notes. This is very valuable help for any instrumentalist or singer. Small movable pieces are also included – a different color has been used for naming each of the seven alphabetical letters – A, B, C, D, E, F, G – which are the names of the musical sounds. Their use gives the hand and the eye a feeling of their relationship. Treble, bass, and C clefs are provided as well as small black and white symbols, both for pitch and for time. It must be stressed that Color Staff does not imply any relationship between sounds and color, but is merely used to link the position of a sound on an instrument to its pitch name and written symbol.

Patterns

Music is essentially composed of patterns – endless different kinds of patterns. The use of Color Staff's separate different colored and named pieces is invaluable for identification of these patterns – for example:

1. the relationship – position of a named musical sound with its place on the staff
2. the repetition of a sound at different pitches
3. the pattern of scales
4. their key signatures
5. intervals
6. chords and their inversions

The material provides an experience of the feeling "within information." It is the means whereby detail can be clarified and an awareness created of "what I was talking about" by putting the learner in touch with facts.

"I think the idea is excellent ... fixing the symbols in the child's imagination as it does. It is useful to have clean staves which, like the blackboard, can be experimented with, and notes put on and off. It is also an excellent way of imprinting the different clefs on the learner's mind."
YEHUDI MENUHIN, K.B.E.

THE COLORS HELP THE EYE TO
ESTABLISH THE RELATIONSHIP
BETWEEN THE NOTES

THE MUSICAL
CLEFS

Conscious control and released and relaxed
awareness allows the musician to express
himself fully through his instrument.

CASE STUDY

Glen Inanga
Piano Student

I am a postgraduate student at the Royal Academy of Music in London studying piano. I have had 21 Alexander Technique lessons, which have been invaluable in my development as a musician.

I first heard of the Alexander Technique seven years ago and realized the potential benefits of the Technique, which included getting the most out of the instrument using least effort. This explained more in context why things worked the way they did. For a long time I had been trying to force the sound out of my instrument and in the process did harmful things to my body. I am also beginning to learn that the technique is akin to a lifetime investment where learning to use the body in the right way in our everyday chores minimizes those problems in the stages of our lives when back pains (for example) begin to crop up. This investment is even more important for me as a musician, since playing an instrument really involves a lot of intense hours of practice.

In our training as pianists, most of the emphasis is on how to play the instrument, and sometimes this is at the risk of misusing our bodies, especially when long, intense hours of practice are involved. Lying down on my back for five minutes after a couple of intense hours of practice is always helpful in heightening the awareness of the relationship between the neck and the back, growing along the spine with the back widening. I find this helps my whole body to "breathe" by opening up previously "cramped" positions which come from bad posture, etc.

After an Alexander Technique lesson, my body experiences a certain lightness in feeling as if it were "uncramped." Before an important recital recently, I had the privilege of having an Alexander Technique lesson in the morning of the same day of the recital. This really proved useful, as it helped me to feel a certain feeling of unity with the instrument, the seat, the floor below me, and above all with the music I was playing. Some have characterized my playing as being rather effortless, particularly in the more physically demanding repertoire. This I can attribute to the principles of the Alexander Technique.

It is my ultimate aim to apply the Technique to the intricacies of the piano which I know will come over a long period of time, but I strongly feel that concentrating for several hours with the most efficient use of our bodies can only yield great results; this way we get the most out of our instruments of expression (ourselves).

PLAYING WIND INSTRUMENTS
TESS MILLER

Every action, whether opening your instrument case, putting your music on the stand, or playing a phrase on the oboe should be initiated, maintained, and completed with ease and freedom.

Habits with which we play begin with the way we put the oboe together. Therefore it is important to observe yourself as you take out a reed or assemble your oboe. Your thoughts about the forthcoming concert, the difficult musical passages involved, and the fact that you wish you had a better reed will manifest physically, causing you to stiffen and use more tension than necessary.

Before playing, give yourself a moment to check that you have made a connection with your feet on the floor and acknowledge that the ground is supporting you and that you are in balance.

Then give your directions. Ask for your neck to be free so your head can go forward and up ... you will then be able to breathe more freely and efficiently, and your body will have at its command all it needs to control the breath and produce the sound you want. It is only when you are out of balance and have lost the connection with the floor that you have to use unnecessary muscular tension.

Similarly, if you are sitting to play, see that the chair is high enough for your thighs to be parallel with the floor (thigh and calf should form a right angle with the knee). Again acknowledge the contact of your feet with the floor, and of your sitting bones with the chair. The floor is supporting both you and the chair. Never sit on one of those plastic molded chairs with a sloping back seat. Before starting to play, be aware of the natural tidal flow of your breathing. Extend your field of awareness to take in your surroundings. This includes your audience. As you are about to play, see that you bring your oboe to your face and not your face to your oboe.

Check this movement in a mirror. It may feel very strange at first to play without shortening your neck muscles and pulling your head down, and it will probably take a little time to cultivate this new and improved use of yourself. But persevere; the dividends are enormous.

Gentle breath of yours my sails must fill.
WILLIAM SHAKESPEARE: *THE TEMPEST*

The guiding hands of the teacher prevent any unnecessary effort in breath production.

CASE STUDY

Tess Miller
*Alexander Teacher and
International Oboist*

I have been a professional oboist all my life, playing both as a soloist and in chamber orchestras. Since I was a teenager, I had suffered from a low back problem. By the time I was in my forties, it was starting to interfere with my work. Sitting for long periods in the orchestra was painful, and I had difficulty carrying my suitcase and instrument on tour. The manager of one of the London chamber orchestras for which I played was herself an Alexander Teacher. I was reluctant to make time for Alexander lessons, but in the end she persuaded me to have a trial lesson. I emerged from the initial lesson a changed being. I floated home on the No. 9 bus, and this extraordinary feeling of physical lightness and freedom persisted for several hours afterward. I continued having regular lessons that proved to be invaluable. They not only helped my back problem, they also gave me insight into the way I reacted to the stress of my profession. Being a musician makes tough demands on one, both physically and psychologically. Through the Alexander Technique I am discovering how my "use" affects my functioning.

Over the years I had acquired poor habits of the use of myself when playing the oboe (i.e. pulling my head and neck forward and down and tensing my shoulders). This had a knock-on effect on my breath control, my ability to articulate the oboe reed quickly with the tip of my tongue, and also the way I responded to "producing the goods" in a concert or when the red light was on in a recording session. As a musician you have to "get it right now." So there is huge incentive to "end-gain" at all costs. I noticed, even when I was thinking about making my oboe reeds, that I was holding my breath and bracing my knees back! This path of discovering how to play with better "use" is an ongoing process, and it is a very exciting one. The Alexander Technique has opened up a new dimension for me, both in my playing and with my oboe teaching. I have also trained to become an Alexander teacher. By inhibition (a means of quickening my observation) and direction, not only am I more at ease with myself, but there is an enhanced freedom in my sound. I have a wider field of awareness that includes my audience. Hitherto my reaction to an audience was to block it off. I am beginning to learn how to be in response to all that is going on, without reacting in my old habitual pattern, which was all too often driven by anxiety and fears, and which resulted in finding myself physically pulled down and mentally less alert. There are moments when I and the oboe are no longer two separate entities. We are a unified resonating whole, participating with the music and being in communication with the audience. I had had tastes of this expanded state before I encountered the Alexander Technique, but I know that the Technique provides a key, a sure means of entry into this sense of being in the moment, and it is just as true for everyday living as it is for playing a musical instrument.

Try not to hold your breath when you put your oboe together.

Be sure your thighs are parallel with the floor and you are sitting on your sitting bones.

Bring your instrument to your mouth. Do not pull yourself down onto your instrument.

VOICE
ROBERT MACDONALD

Speak the speech, I pray you, as I pronounc'd it to you, trippingly on the tongue, but if you mouth it, as many of our players do, I had as live the town-crier spoke my lines. Nor do not saw the air too much with your hand, thus, but use all gently, for in the very torrent, tempest, and, as I may say, whirlwind of your passion, you must acquire and beget a temperance that may give it smoothness.

WILLIAM SHAKESPEARE: *HAMLET*

Most people are born with an outstanding vocal instrument. Babies make extraordinary sounds, notable for their power, resonance, and emotional variety. We would expect that as we grow in stature and strength the voice would mirror this development. Unfortunately, this is not always the case, and often the aging process brings with it a decline of vocal performance.

When the voice is allowed to operate as a reflex process, it will be free. Once the intention to speak is

Most babies have excellent natural vocal dexterity

present, the vocal mechanism is designed to make all the necessary preparations automatically. If we decide to carry out our intention to speak, the body is poised to carry out our intention – the energized breath, the working position of the larynx, the activation of the vocal folds, and the sympathetic activity of the resonators take place in a complex and beautifully coordinated way.

Alexander made a fundamental discovery about how human beings limit their vocal potential. His perceptive observation of how he used himself in performance led to the realization that his vocal problem reflected an overall pattern of misuse, and overcoming the problem required an evolution of physical and mental awareness. Because the voice is suspended in the body, its free activity depends on the postural mechanisms working efficiently; any inefficiency of the postural body will impose limitations on the voice. The Alexander Technique, by bringing about natural body support, gives the voice the support it needs and the chance to work freely. It then helps us to move into energized activity while avoiding any interference that limits it.

The release of the breathing reflex is fundamental to vocal freedom and resonance. A bell, once struck by an initial attack, will resonate until the sound gradually dies away unless something interferes with the bell, e.g. a hand. Resonance is a process of resounding, allowing sound to sound again. The voice works because of an interaction between breath flow, vibration, and the open spaces of the resonators. The role of the voice teacher is to encourage this interactive flow, and to help pupils recognize the primary role of their upright posture in creating the natural support for this to happen. Postural awareness leads to a greater sense of the gripping and constriction that obstruct the free flow necessary to sound with fullness and prominence.

Speaking in a large space tends to frighten us. We become anxious about what is to be said and to whom, and how to fill the space with sound. We try to project the voice. Projection is not helpful because it suggests that we need to force the voice out of the body. Light projects, but sound resonates. The old singing masters encouraged us to bring sound back into the body if we wished to fill a larger space. Only by realizing our full internal space, and using that to engage the voice, will we be able to communicate and fill a large external space with powerful, resonant, free-flowing sound.

The Alexander Technique increases our muscular awareness and helps the performer to make choices about "how" they do what they do. It helps to make the distinction between the essential energy needed for voice and the tensions that limit our vocal potential, leading not only to an increase in power, flexibility, and range, but to an "openness" on every level. Expressing emotion with honesty, clarity, and variety is essential in the vocal arts. In everyday life, the expression of emotion is often accompanied by extreme muscular contraction. In performance, excessive tension in the performer can have the curious effect of blocking the emotion or of making it appear indulgent. The ability to feel the difference between muscular energy and inappropriate tension helps performers to release into emotional expression. It helps them to discard what is unnecessary in performance, and to develop the confidence and simplicity that are the basis of true communication.

Resonance

After sound has been made by the action of the breath stream and the vibration of the vocal folds, it can be modified and enhanced by the resonators giving it body and audibility – or general resonance. It is the inherent size, general shape, and number of apertures (the large ratio of pharyngeal to oral cavity area is a distinguishing feature of the male vocal tract), and the quality and density of the walls of the pharynx, nose, and mouth that will determine the sound frequencies and the unique acoustical patterns that give each voice its distinctive quality. The resonators can be classed as subglottic, consisting of the thoracic (the lungs, as a large air space, have their own fundamental tone) and tracheal cavities, and supraglottic (consisting of the pharyngeal, oral, and nasal cavities, and the buccal cavities, i.e. the air space between lips, teeth, and cheeks). The subglottic resonators provide air spaces that are set into sympathetic vibration with the vocal folds and act as universal resonators. The principal resonators of the voice are the supraglottic resonators.

FRONTAL
SINUS

SPHENOIDAL
SINUS

NASAL
CAVITY

ORAL
CAVITY

PHARYNGEAL
CAVITY

LARYNX

Good vocal performance demands full attention to mind, body, and spirit.

Breathing

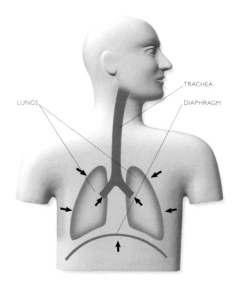

When the brain recognizes that an inbreath is required, the diaphragm is drawn down, expanding the lung space and causing air to fill the lungs.

During expiration, the diaphragm relaxes and returns to its customary domed shape, reducing the lung space in preparation for the next inbreath.

The respiratory center of the brain monitors the level of oxygen/carbon dioxide in the lungs. When more breath is required, an impulse is sent to the diaphragm to contract, causing it to flatten and descend. It presses on the abdominal viscera, which drop down and eventually resist the downward movement. The abdomen then acts as a fixed point from which the diaphragm, assisted by the external intercostal muscles, elevates the lower ribs. The lungs, which are attached to the ribcage, are expanded by this movement and the chest is enlarged.

Due to the previous expiration and the subsequent expansion of the lungs by the diaphragm, atmospheric pressure is now greater than lung pressure. That imbalance is quickly adjusted by an automatic, reflex intake of air. The student must be aware that tensions, such as pulling down, sniffing, and gasping, interfere with an effortless intake of breath.

During inspiration, the action of the diaphragm on the viscera and abdominal muscles causes an increase of intra-abdominal pressure. During expiration, this natural buildup of pressure, together with other elastic forces such as the muscular tendons of the chest wall,

the lungs, and the torque of the ribs, can decrease the volume of the thoracic cavity independently of any voluntary muscular contraction. This natural shifting of pressures is the basis of high-performance breathing, and it is important that students experience, early in their voice training, the ease and power of this involuntary, elastic cycle.

During expiration the diaphragm needs to relax and rise fully to its domelike shape in readiness for the next inspiration. It is essential that the full stature of the body is maintained, as any degree of "pulling down" or "collapse" will prevent the full rise of the diaphragm, with a consequent imperfect inspiration when it is next activated.

In normal breathing the length of inspiration and expiration are almost equal. When speaking or singing, the length of expiration is longer than the length of the inspiration. Students tend to interfere with their breathing reflex in their desire to extend the length of their outbreath and accelerate the speed of their inbreath. This interference will be visible in the excessive tension that they use to hold the body and control the breath.

CASE STUDY

VOICE STUDENT
The London Academy of
Music and Dramatic Art (LAMDA)

Before I started having Alexander lessons, my muscular tension had a negative impact on the performance, the emotion, everything, on the voice. You know you have these tensions, but I think of them as disconnected from the performance, that you are giving this great performance and there are these tensions, but they are not important, whereas in fact they are affecting everything – the vocal quality, the clarity of thought, and the truthfulness of my emotions.

When I did the speech, I did feel a change about half-way through, and that was linked to a forward-and-up head direction which rooted me more and meant that I felt more with the speech. My voice felt very different,

much more solid and rooted and how I wanted it to be … And more elastic as well – I felt more able to just do something if I wanted to do it. What was interesting about doing it in the mirror was that … objectifying yourself you are less stern on yourself so you allowed yourself time, like when you watch someone else and you say, "Just take your time, don't rush, don't push yourself"– I was able to treat myself with that distance and not push myself or apologize for myself, and the other thing that I noticed was that through watching myself, I was able to spot when things went into a direction that I didn't want them to go in terms of tensing and pushing and immediately apply conscious inhibition, relocate, and start again, so that on each breath really there was a new opportunity, a new starting point to go again, and it didn't just feel like the first word of the speech was a roller-coaster you get on; if it is a bumpy ride, tough luck, you got on that seat and you can't change once you are on it.

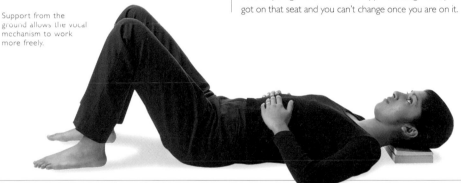

Support from the ground allows the vocal mechanism to work more freely.

Practicing expiration by blowing the air out allows effortless inspiration.

Releasing
Your Voice

Voice work begins with good breathing. Efficient breathing relies on efficient posture, being able to breathe out and then allow the air into the body without loss of length or width. Bracing up like a soldier or collapsing down like a deflated balloon will disturb natural breathing and interfere with your voice.

Practicing in semi-supine position is good because it helps you to build up the experience of maintaining your full size during vocal exercises. The back in contact with the ground gives support to your body, reducing the tendency to collapse or pull down. The contact with the ground gives you more body feedback, helping you to be aware of unnecessary rigidity or effort, particularly any tendency to retract the head.

Lie in semi-supine (see Lying Down, Semi-supine, page 78), remembering that this position allows your

muscles to release and grow in stature. Any attempt to force or accelerate change will be counterproductive and interfere with your voice (see End-gaining, page 35). As you lie on the floor with your head supported by the correct height of books, place your hands on your lower ribs. This will allow you to observe the spontaneous changes in your breathing. Now close your mouth and breathe out and in through your nose. If you continue to apply inhibition and direction, air will come in and out through your nose and your breathing will gradually become slower and deeper.

Extend the length of the out-breath so that you slightly increase the amount of breath that you expel from the body. This will stimulate more air to come in. Now when you breathe out, blow the air through your lips. Close your mouth and breathe in through the nose. Repeat the exhalation three times and then stop.

At the end of the above sequence, it is important that you apply the principles of inhibition and direction, and

Lying down enables you to become aware of the tensions that interfere with your vocal freedom.

Using the Mirror

Stand in front of a full-length mirror. Breathe out on the "fff" sound and close your mouth to allow the breath back in through the nose. Repeat three times. When you have completed the exercise, observe yourself in the mirror and ask, "Did I stiffen my neck and pull my body down during the procedure? Did I collapse during exhalation? Did I tighten my neck and lift my shoulders to breathe in?" Avoiding these patterns establishes a basis that will help your voice work freely and energetically.

re-establish full contact with the floor through the nine points of support. As you direct your attention in this way it may help you to answer the question, "In the exercise, did I stiffen my neck and pull my head back?" Being open to this feedback from the body at the end of an exercise is crucial for the growth and development of your voice. It will help you to become aware of the unconscious tensions and muscular patterns that interfere with your voice production. Then you are in a position to avoid them.

In a moment you can try the breathing-out exercise again, but before you do consider the phrase "conscious involuntary exhalation." Conscious exhalation means that you are aware of the importance of breathing out in order to allow the air back into the body. Lowering the volume of air in the lungs in this way stimulates the breathing reflex. Conscious exhalation also means that you are aware of how important it is to release to your full length through the exercise, and that you place primary importance on maintaining your full free stature through voice exercises.

Involuntary exhalation means that you are allowing the out-breath to happen. It is possible for the movement of the ribcage to take care of itself in response to your simple decision to exhale. Provided that you don't collapse or pull down, the thought to breathe out will generate an easy, powerful, free-flowing out-breath. When emphasis is placed on the direct muscular manipulation of the ribcage, you can become too concerned about how the ribs should move, and try to achieve the "correct" movement of the rib-cage. Concentrating on maintaining even pressure, or sustaining the breath through a long phrase, can be counterproductive in the early stages of voice work, because it interferes with the inherent ease and spontaneity of the ribs.

When you explore a way of working that leads you to experience the inherent ease, elasticity, and power of your ribcage, you allow the movement to respond to your decision to breathe out while maintaining your full length. You are giving the movement permission to happen, rather than controlling it.

Now try the exercise again. As you allow yourself to maintain contact with the ground, breathe out on the blowing sound. The formation of the lips provides just the right amount of resistance so that you don't expel the air all at once. This gentle resistance will help to give you the confidence to let your ribs go, and to experience the spontaneous power of the movement when you let it happen.

The ribcage naturally moves to sustain the breath if you do not interfere with it.

Shut your lips and allow the air back in through your nose. Repeat this cycle three times. Then stop, give your directions, and gradually re-establish contact with the ground. Mastering this basic exercise will give you a foundation that will improve every aspect of your voice work. Repeat the breathing-out exercise, but on the third exhalation, instead of blowing, hum.

It is the free-flowing breath that eventually becomes sound, and the more you adopt the process of ease and release as opposed to contraction and effort, the more you are establishing the foundation for vocal excellence. Becoming aware of and preventing wrong habits helps you to get the most out of your voice. This means learning to recognize the muscular tensions that are unnecessary and then learning how to prevent them freely. The time we spend at the end of an exercise is crucial because it is taking the necessary time to receive the feedback from the body. By listening to the feedback, we can begin to recognize the difference between energy necessary for vocal expression and when we are creating inappropriate tension.

SINGING

Singing is so fine a thing
I wish all men would learn to sing

JOHN CLARE

There cannot be any sound where there is no
movement or percussion of the air. There cannot
be any percussion of the air where there is no
instrument. There cannot be any instrument
without a body.

LEONARDO DA VINCI, NOTEBOOKS

Before we developed the art of either oral or written
language to communicate with one another, we sang
imitatively, echoing the melodies heard in nature.
These expressions are the deepest feelings of
humankind that cut across nationalities, class, and
age. They soothe us and stir us up, reduce us to tears
and sustain us. "Music hath charms to still the
savage beast."

We are designed to make sound. The very word
"person" comes from the Latin *persona*, meaning "that
through which sound passes." It refers to the
megaphone mask worn by actors in Greco-Roman
drama. The Greeks believed that the voice was the soul
escaping from the body. The Greek word *psyche*,
meaning "soul," has the same root as *psychen*, meaning
"to breathe," and the word *pneuma*, meaning "spirit"
also means wind.

There is a deep and intimate connection between
the breath and the psyche. We could say we truly
express ourselves through sound.

Full expression of the voice is possible if the body is stable and balanced.

The Valsalva Maneuver

The epiglottis is a flap of skin that folds over the top of your windpipe to prevent food from being breathed into the lungs; it closes when you make a great effort. When you want to push very hard on something, or lift a big weight, you often grunt. (Remember the noise that some tennis players make as they serve?) What you are doing is filling your lungs with air and then shutting the epiglottis. This allows you to build up pressure inside the lungs to make your chest hard and firm. Then it is much easier to push or lift. When the epiglottis is shut, you may be able to lift a heavy weight or perform a strenuous action, but you will not be able to sing.

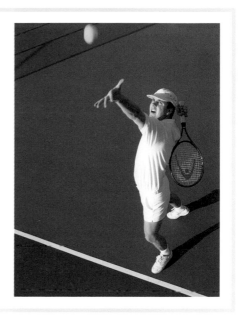

Anatomy and Physiology of Singing

When we sing, we use the whole vocal mechanism in a heightened way – the amount of emotional and muscular energy needed to vocalize increases. The muscles of breathing, the muscles that suspend the larynx, the muscles that open and close the throat, and the muscles of articulation attach into the overall framework of the body.

For these muscles to function freely and to work together in a coordinated fashion, the body must lengthen in stature. This lengthening creates an antagonistic pull in the body musculature and increases the opportunity to use energy effectively. There is a degree of misunderstanding about how this antagonism works. Take the example of the steering wheel of your car. When you turn it, are you pulling it or are you pushing it? When you pull it down on one side, you are pushing it up on the other. It is all one – push–pull – constantly adjusting the intercostal muscle tension, the relaxation of the diaphragm, and decreasing volume of the thoracic cavity leading to exhaling air from the lungs. These adjustments then affect the distribution of tension in the larynx.

The stability of the upper chest should be maintained at all times when singing.

Everybody Sings

When you come to sing, the relevant muscles know what to do. A baby "sings" before she speaks. The first cooing sounds and "Ah's" that you hear are experiments which she makes for hours on end, listening to the sounds she can make. Eventually she begins to formulate meaningful sounds and the "Ah's" become "Mama," or a similar sound to which the mother responds. The connection between a sound and a person is forged. The infant lets her mother know her needs through sound.

Babies sing before they learn to speak

We sing first – song lives in the hind brain, the old part in evolutionary terms.

Singers often fall into the habit of using too much breath to sing. Of course you need breath, but so often

A jazz singer employs a special quality of breathiness.

the initial intake is miscalculated. A particular relationship between the pressure of breath and the vocal folds is necessary to create a beautiful sound, and the lengthening of the stature creates the overall framework that the voice needs to work well. Overbreathing disrupts that interaction. You will know when you are overbreathing – you stiffen your neck and shorten and narrow your body.

The actual sound of your voice is affected by breath. It is possible to push too much breath through the glottis and give an audibly breathy or even husky quality to the voice. If you do this, you will be wasting air and not be able to sing and sustain long phrases. The exhalation will be more like a sigh that escapes unavoidably. When the quality of breathiness is required in the voice such as for jazz and blues singing,

then there is no problem. But when this vocal quality is not wanted, it causes great distress for singers. They are advised to "get onto their breath," but often lack the ability to know how to do this. The Alexander Technique helps to reduce this habit by connecting the voice and the breath *(see Whispered "Ah's," page 84)*.

The tendency to stiffen the legs causes problems for singers. When this happens, the feet are flattened onto the floor and the "Bubbling Spring," the arch, is tightened. As the legs relate muscularly to the root of the diaphragm, there is a subsequent tightening in this muscle that produces a restricted sound. Instead of the voice being on the wheel of the breath, it seems to be trapped in the spokes. When the legs and feet are freely connected to the back and diaphragm, the voice can come like a fountain.

When I hear a voice that is not coming out fully, energized and present, then I know there is nothing coming up from the source.

DAVID CAREY, SENIOR VOICE LECTURER,
CENTRAL SCHOOL OF SPEECH AND DRAMA, LONDON

Bel Canto

Bel canto, which means "beautiful song," was the particular art of singing and composing that flourished throughout the 17th and 18th centuries in Italy. It demanded from the singer an ability to communicate genuine emotion musically and precisely, spanning a vocal range of three octaves. Great attention was paid to verbal diction and refinement of tone. It was the flexibility of the sound and the quality of the timbres combined with the beautiful, expressive sound that made bel canto unique.

The Suspensory Mechanism of the Larynx

The larynx is suspended by a muscular network that stretches the larynx in four different directions. These muscles operate in opposition to each other. The antagonistic stretch brings about the "suspension" of the larynx and makes the proper closure of the vocal folds possible. Unlocking the voice depends on the lengthened stretch of these opposing forces. If the suspensory mechanism is functioning poorly, then it will be difficult to achieve a "low-lying" larynx, and inappropriate effort will be required in order to sing. If we observe the attachment points of the suspensory network, it is clear that the balance of the head and lengthening and widening in stature are crucial in bringing about the antagonistic stretch. An abundant supply of nerves allow the movement of the larynx to be controlled very precisely.

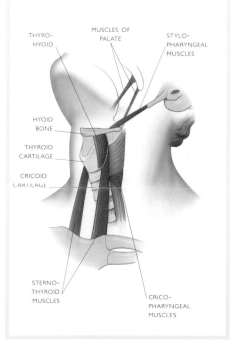

THYRO-HYOID

MUSCLES OF PALATE

STYLO-PHARYNGEAL MUSCLES

HYOID BONE

THYROID CARTILAGE

CRICOID CARTILAGE

STERNO-THYROID MUSCLES

CRICO-PHARYNGEAL MUSCLES

HIDEMI HATADA
Opera Singer and Alexander Teacher

When you don't have any idea what Alexander Technique is, you tend to react to it with, "I am a musician. I do not need to change!" Because you might misunderstand that Alexander Technique is a kind of way to find out or treat something you do wrong. It is not true.

It is to deal with awareness of what you are doing unconsciously. Breathing, producing voice, movement while performing, how you react to music, text, acting, or other musicians you are singing with, even how you use your creative sense. Once you realize how you do these, then your mind and body are getting freer and more flexible to whatever you want, and your performance, singing or playing on the stage, is coming alive. If you could feel all of that, Alexander Technique would be very tasty!

Suggestions for Singing Practice

- Stop any immediate response to prepare to sing. This can be very difficult because as soon as you hear the accompanist's first notes, you are ready to go for it.
- Give the new directions that allow you to stand at your full height by letting your head nod forward in order to go up. Do not look up for guidance; be musically prepared and you will not need help.
- Do some whispered "Ah's."
- Gently and easily hum with your mouth closed.
- Begin to hum and then open your mouth and keep humming so the sound stays inside.
- Hum, then open your mouth while still humming, then sing "Ah" as a sustained note.
- Begin to sing, but consciously consider how you are singing. Stop if you find yourself going back to your old habits of overpreparing and tightening.
- Try not to anticipate problems, and do not allow the high notes to make you frightened and think you need to push.
- Enjoy it!

PUBLIC SPEAKING AND PRESENTATION SKILLS

ANNE FREEMAN

Standing up in front of a group of people and offering something of yourself – talent, skill, expertise – is nerve-racking, however small the group and however experienced the performer. There is no exception to this. Any performer who claims not to feel at least some degree of anxiety is one who does not perform to the best of his or her ability.

Those who have to present information in the course of their work are performers, just like any actor or singer. Usually, in career terms, there is just as much riding on their performance. The business audience, like the theater or opera audience, will generally include competitive peers or aspirants, judgmental superiors or observers, as well as actual or potential customers. The basics of preparation are similar: selection of material; learning; rehearsal. The audience receives a similar sequence of impressions – appearance, voice, and ultimately, the text. There are sometimes even props to deal with, such as the dreaded overhead projector or the latest computerized gadget! So presentation skills can rightly be equated with performance skills, and presentation nerves with stage fright.

In teaching presentation and voice, I find the Alexander Technique central to every aspect of working with a wide variety of students requiring this kind of help, from the most senior in management or the professions to the newest trainee.

The Technique informs the essentials of posture, breath, vocal quality, physical dexterity, and efficient and assured movement, as well as being linked at a deeper and more subtle level to the functioning and accessibility of the personality.

Every performance, like every individual, contains two major elements, the external and the internal – how I seem and how I feel. The Alexander Technique underlies both and unites them.

When the neck is free, the head forward and up, the back long and wide, and the breathing low and efficient, the audience will see a poised stance and easy movement. They will hear an attractive, well-placed voice inspiring confidence. They will be able to relax and take in the words, without worrying about whether the performer is going to cope.

Equally important, the Technique supports the internal element. When the body is correctly used and the voice is agile and well articulated; when we know we can inhibit our immediate panic or excitement responses and so remember our text and deliver it honestly; when we can take the time we need to answer even the most difficult questions appropriately, then we can get out of our own way and make a real connection with the audience. The goal in convincing an audience is for the internal and external selves to become the same. When the mind, body, and voice are saying the same thing, the audience knows that we are telling the truth.

The Alexander Technique cannot affect the quality of the message, but it has proved itself fundamental to developing the quality of the messenger.

The Alexander Technique allows you to present your subject and yourself with poise.

Stage Fright

We have all experienced the symptoms of stage fright or performance anxiety – sweating, trembling, nausea, and diarrhea. A certain amount of arousal and even anxiety which produces the adrenalin flow can make for a better performance, but too much anxiety can be debilitating. There are a number of factors that can influence the likelihood of how we respond to public performance. Some people are naturally more nervous than others. Some situations are more demanding than others: an important audition or public performance, some pieces of music and dramatic roles, are more difficult than others. If performers are underprepared for an engagement, stage fright always results.

It is useful to consider the difference between performance anxiety, which tends to be debilitating, and performance excitement, which is the natural way of generating the necessary energy to give a good performance. Performance anxiety involves an excessive increase in muscle tension that shortens and narrows the body stature; the performer will find himself struggling to breathe.

Alexander organized performances of *Hamlet* and *The Merchant of Venice* at the Old Vic Theatre in London using inexperienced actors. Contrary to expectations, they did not suffer from stage fright even without the services of a prompter.

My friends and critics naturally anticipated a wonderful exhibition of "stage fright" on the evening of the first performance, but as a matter of fact not one of my young students had the least apprehension of that terror. By the time they were ready to appear, the idea of "stage fright" was one that seemed to them the merest absurdity. It may be said that they did not understand what was meant by such a condition. And this, although I would not allow a prompter on the nights of the public performances.

F.M. ALEXANDER:
MAN'S SUPREME INHERITANCE

MICHELLE KENT
Studio Administrator,
Royal College of Music

When I commenced lessons in Alexander Technique, I had high expectations of the results I wished to achieve; these have been surpassed in a very short time.

The most obvious benefit is the feeling of being able to cope and to stand on my own two feet, providing clearer focus in decision-making, greater self-confidence and self-control, leading to a much calmer approach to everything. I have lost the sense of panic I used to get when faced with more than I thought I could cope with. As a result of this new-found security, I feel I am able to provide more support to others.

I have also noticed a marked improvement in my voice, so that I am singing with greater ease (especially high notes, with which I had problems previously). Another consequence is the release of creativity, allowing freedom of thought and opening other channels for relaxation (music, drawing, and writing). Taking part in a jazz music summer school (singing) was, for me, a real test of these new skills and one which proved just how valuable they are. New experiences such as this are often daunting and unnerving, but I was able to turn my fast day of dread into a fun and exciting week of learning new skills (vocal improvisation especially) and performing in the club each night without tension in my neck and shoulders.

The increased energy, sense of direction, and inner strength gained have changed my outlook on life dramatically.

PAINTING
ELIZA ANDREWS

The difference between a bad and a good drawing could be said to be the difference between a copy and a personal interpretation of the subject. The Alexander Technique can help the physical activity that leads to the creative activity that produces a painting or drawing.

Painting is the equation of:
1. Concept
2. Medium (i.e. the material used)
3. Human body

So often the use of the human body is taken for granted until trouble occurs in the form of pain. Exceptions include Chinese brush-painting and calligraphy, in which body technique is appreciated.

The concept is an intellectual factor, assisted by maximizing the potential of the human body for a particular purpose. When using an easel or painting murals, you have an upright surface at some distance. When doing illustrations or calligraphy, you have a sloping surface close to you.

The medium you use can vary and requires different conditions. If the painting is large-scale, it is often easier to work on the floor. If the paint is very wet, you will need to work on a horizontal surface.

The human body is the implement you use to draw and paint *(see Handwriting, page 70)*. The natural radius of the wrist, elbow, and arm renders the drawing of a perfect circle possible.

Drawing Circles

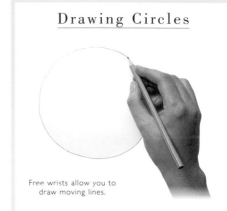

Free wrists allow you to draw moving lines.

If you experience difficulty in drawing free continuous lines, check that you are not holding your breath, stiffening your wrists, and generally pulling down.

It is important to be aware of how you are holding your brush as well as what you are painting.

If you take time to set up your equipment properly, you will save yourself undue muscular tension.

Good Design

When drawing, the line you create follows the circular idea and is curved. In order to make it straight, pressure is needed to push the line upward. As this happens, drawing is no longer a released action, and tension creeps in as concentration increases. This can lead to the habit of holding your breath and hunching your shoulders.

Posture is an important consideration in this skill/art. One of the first decisions is whether to stand or to sit to paint. A second consideration is what distance is required for you to be able to assess your work and get a clear view of the whole.

When sitting, you have the possibility of a close-up focus (e.g. calligraphy, miniature painting, some illustration work). The radius of the whole arm is limited in this position, so the danger of hunching the shoulders and coming down in front needs to be recognized and avoided.

When standing using an easel, you have the possibility of the whole radius of the arm, ideal for releasing the shoulder. The danger in this position is that as you tire, you tend to pull down into the hips. Standing to paint requires a good deal of stamina.

There is a great diversity of equipment available for the painter, but often it is not easily accessible to the beginner outside art school. Necessity is the mother of invention. When you are aware of the height of the work, surfaces you need, you can put a brick at one end of your kitchen table so your drawing board rests on an appropriate slope or put two crates to raise it to the height of a designer's work table.

> Height of table top: approximately
> 28 inches/70 cm from ground.
> Gradient of slope: approximately
> $3^1/_2$ inches in 12 inches/9 cm in 30 cm.

The Victorian sloping desk was better than the flat tables of today.

Working on the floor on a large surface can be physically demanding, often leading to the bent-back position. Releasing from the hands and knees (crawling) position into painting activity can help. Take breaks to get up and give your directions.

> Height of designer's work-top:
> 36–40 inches/90–100 cm from ground.

It has an adjustable slope from horizontal to near-vertical with a choice of standing or using a high stool. Like the easel, this is ideal as it allows adjustments to be made easily, and sitting and standing can be alternated. Some pieces of equipment seem to lead to problems. The sketching stool and board can encourage a cramped position and movement. A folding easel and stool chair are more appropriate for sketching.

If you choose to sit while painting, make sure you maintain your full height.

If you collapse down in front, you will restrict your breathing and your dexterity.

SPORT AND RECREATION
CONSCIOUS EXERCISE

THE PRACTICE OF exercising to build muscle and lose weight is a modern one. For the ancient Greeks exercise was a vital part of daily life, and it was the responsibility of a good citizen to keep himself in good physical condition. Exercise was not an exclusively physical activity, however, but seen as a way of developing the spiritual side of life, a practice of allowing mind and body to work together in harmonious perfection. Mindless exercise would have had no place in the system.

Balance is essential when skateboarding.

What (he lacked) was a conscious and proper recognition of the right uses of the parts of his muscular mechanism, since while he uses such parts wrongly, the performance of physical exercises will only increase the defects...while his own consciousness of the act performed and the means and uses of his muscular mechanism will remain unaltered. Therefore before he attempts any form of physical development he must discover... what his defects are...

F.M. ALEXANDER: MAN'S SUPREME INHERITANCE

Alexander questioned the modern attitude to exercise of trying to "get fit" – "Fit for what?" was his question. He was concerned that people were not paying enough attention to how they exercised and were in danger of doing themselves more harm than good. He observed that in exercising their muscles, they were creating a lot of inappropriate tension and lowering their awareness of their body. He believed that this way of exercising could increase physical defects and make people less able to manage their bodies easily and efficiently.

The scientific study of exercise has confirmed that, although a certain amount of exercise helps to keep us healthy, when we overexercise we may be suppressing rather than enhancing the immune system. The idea of achieving peak performance by exercising the body into exhaustion and then letting it recover is being questioned by both sports experts and scientists. It is not just a matter of how much you do, but how efficiently you work. This means that you learn to pay attention to "how" you exercise. Perhaps you have experienced occasions when the harder you tried, the less you achieved. Conscious exercise encourages you to cultivate effortlessness. The expert makes it look easy.

Learning to exercise consciously involves paying attention to the signals from your body. How you use your body and how you breathe are the two primary indicators, giving you the feedback that will help you to know the amount of exercise that helps you to reduce stress and the amount that could lead to you over-exercising and actually creating stress.

Although exercise leads to increased activity in your muscles, conscious exercise encourages you to maintain good use throughout dynamic activity. As soon as you find yourself unable to maintain your directions in the activity, your body is telling you that you are exceeding its present capacity for easy dynamism.

The second indicator is the effectiveness of your breathing. It is often thought acceptable to stretch the body to its maximum capacity. By doing this you could end up gasping the air in through the mouth. An alternative perspective on proper exercise asks how active you can be without having to resort to mouth breathing.

Exercise can release the latent stored energy within us.

Conscious Exercise

Conscious exercise encourages you to pay attention to:

1. PREPARATION.

2. FEEDBACK DURING PERFORMANCE:

- Listening to the body: fixed or free; expanding or collapsing and/or contracting down.
- Breathing: mouth or nose; easy or excessive effort to breathe in

3. RECOVERY:

- Re-establish your full stature.
- Return to nose breathing.

Before you are able to apply these principles to your preferred sport, you will need to apply them to a simple activity. Try this experiment while out walking in the park.

1. STOP AND THINK ABOUT YOUR PREPARATION:

- Inhibit and give your directions to achieve your full stature.
- Allow the air out and in through the nose.
- Be aware of your environment.

2. START TO WALK:

- Achieve a comfortable speed and rhythm.
- Listen to the feedback your body is giving you, and maintain nose-breathing.
- Increase speed as you continue to be aware of your use and breathing.

3. AS SOON AS YOU BEGIN TO SHORTEN YOUR STATURE AND RESORT TO MOUTH BREATHING, THEN YOU MUST STOP AND RECOVER:

- Stand still.
- Release the shortening muscles and allow your self to lengthen and widen.
- Allow your breathing to recover, breathing out and in through the nose.

Fit for Life

Gradually you will find that you can exert more energy while continuing to maintain good use and efficient breathing. You can then go into a light run, provided that you remain open to the feedback from your self and are prepared to stop and recover when you begin to exceed your body's present capacity. After a while you will find that you start to become mindful of these principles in your day-to-day activities and you will be able to apply them to all your sporting activities. You will have laid the foundation of an exercising process where increased activity means increased well-being.

In competitive events, an athlete is given points for how well the task is performed. In ice skating, ballroom dancing, gymnastics, a top score of ten points may be awarded. High scores come from executing the movement with as few mistakes as possible. The more mistakes, the lower the score. Achieving a high score demands skill and poise, and an understanding of how best to perform the task.

Dynamic posture is posture in motion or in action. Good dynamic posture implies the use of the body or its parts in the simplest and most effective way. For a neuromuscular skeletal performance to be easy and graceful and fulfilling, you need muscle contraction and relaxation, balance, coordination, timing, and rhythm all working together harmoniously.

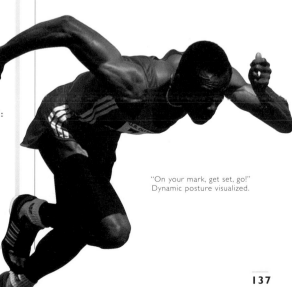

"On your mark, get set, go!"
Dynamic posture visualized.

T'AI CHI CHUAN
FRANK TREMBATH

For centuries, the Martial Arts have been studied as a way of gaining self-discipline of the highest order. Martial means war – not simply with the enemy, but with yourself, conquering your fears and weakness. To become a master demands a high level of training and self-discipline leading to freedom and strength, as well as accuracy. The mastery of self is necessary before any victory can be achieved. This state can be gained only after long years of disciplined study.

"The Saint Points
the Way"

FRANK TREMBATH
*Practitioner of T'ai Chi Chuan
and Alexander Teacher*

T'ai Chi is a soft or internal Chinese martial art, different to the hard or external martial arts such as Karate and T'ae Kwon Do. I have been Studying T'ai Chi for 20 years and the Alexander Technique for 15. Both disciplines put forth very similar ideas. The vocabulary may be different, but the essence of what is being expressed is comparable. During the Alexander lesson the pupil is asked to inhibit the habitual way he uses himself. Before a pupil begins a T'ai Chi Chuan "form" – a series of postures performed in sequence – he is asked to calm himself and empty the mind and "let the head be balanced as if suspended from above." In Alexander Technique this could be "free the neck and let the head go forward and up." When practicing T'ai Chi we should be neither collapsed nor stiff and rigid, and the muscles should be lengthening. Joints and muscles are never locked or held in fixed positions. The postures are constantly changing and are always in balance. To perform T'ai Chi Chuan correctly, a free neck is absolutely essential. Another important similarity is embodied in the concept of end-gaining. Alexander teaches us that it is not the end that requires our attention but the means whereby that end is gained. In T'ai Chi Chuan, the importance is not how many forms or movements we have acquired, but the quality of those movements; not completing a sequence of movements but the means whereby that sequence is completed. The Alexander Technique has given me a greater awareness of my musculature, enabling me to identify overcontracted muscle. My proprioceptive sense has developed, allowing me to sense more accurately the position of my body in space and in relationship to itself. This has given me the basis for a better functioning of the muscular skeletal system and consequent reduction of wear and tear.

"The Snake
Creeps Down"

RIDING A HORSE
DANIEL PEVSNER
FELLOW OF THE BRITISH HORSE SOCIETY

His ears up-pricked, his braided hanging mane,
Upon his compassed crest now stand on end.
His nostrils drink the air – and forth again,
As from a furnace, vapours doth he send.

WILLIAM SHAKESPEARE: *VENUS AND ADONIS*

Humans have ridden horses since the earliest times. The horse has given us both pleasure and service. When we watch riders, we can see a wide range of skills. The ultimate state is when horse and rider seem to merge together and be acting as one. This harmony can be so complete that just a thought from the rider is enough to trigger a response in the horse. The rider has the ability to influence and control the horse through the appropriate use of his own back. This action involves the rider altering the degree of stretch and tension of his spine. He does this very subtly, actually using his back as a working tool that he can activate and adjust at will. When synchronized with the legs and hands, it has a very powerful influence on the horse. A living body cannot be forced to act in a particular manner, at most it can be coaxed into so doing. This principle, which the Alexander Technique persistently reiterates, is the same for people and horses. We have the freedom to choose. The Alexander Technique gives guidance.

Comparison between Animal and Human Movement

The horse's head rotates forward and up at a point just behind the ears, called the poll, while the lower jaw softens. This allows breathing and salivation to happen freely. The horse's neck stretches forward, and up with a slight arch, as the back lengthens and widens. The horse's head leads the body. The head direction allows the neck and back to stretch forward and as a consequence the legs start moving to support the weight. The back is pulsating all the time, and the breathing is regular, giving elasticity and tone to the movement.

What Constitutes a Good Riding Position?

A good riding position is often described as "The Classical Seat." The rider should sit upright so that each part of his body rests on that which is immediately below it, so the effect of the weight of the rider reaches the horse in a vertical manner, through the seat bones *(see Sitting, page 66)*. This position offers:

FOR THE RIDER – security and comfort in the saddle and the ability to guide the horse with ease and efficiency.
FOR THE HORSE – reduction to a minimum of any discomfort that the rider's weight on its back might cause.

This position has to be maintained while the horse is moving simultaneously in the horizontal and vertical directions, curving and moving sideways. This calls for a high degree of firm suppleness in the rider that can blend and absorb pressure while retaining its resilience and ability to recapture its original shape quickly.

Daniel Pevsner on Tippy, owned by M. Rice Edwards, beginning of piaffe.

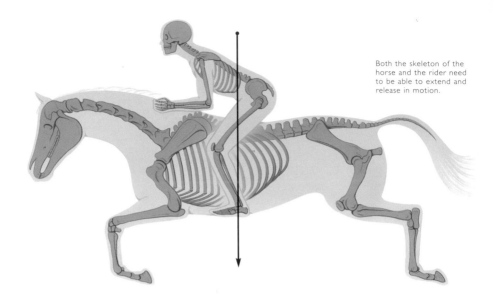

Both the skeleton of the horse and the rider need to be able to extend and release in motion.

The Correct Classical Seat

Compare Alexander Technique seat, spine lengthened, back widened, free working joints, regular breathing, supple body. Weight supported on the seat bones and the tail bone which is cushioned by the buttock muscles.

Chair Seat

Pressure on abdomen, constriction of ribs and diaphragm, reduction in breathing, shoulders raised, chest caved in, upper back rounded, arms stiffened, thighs angled forward.

Forked Seat

Overtense; attempt to achieve "good posture" ("Mountie"), hollowed back, chest lifted, weight forward, tense hands, legs, head pulled back.

WELL BALANCED

CHAIR

FORKED

Charles Harris

Charles Harris – Fellow of the Institute of the Horse; Fellow of Association of British Riding Schools; Fellow of the British Horse Society. He is the first English person to have completed the full three-year training course of the Spanish Riding School in Vienna.

"Correctly controlled movement of the horse's head and neck – combined with the correct use of the rider's body – ensures equine equilibrium and efficiency."

Respiration in Horses

If you watch a horse galloping you will see the rib-cage expand as the legs come underneath the body, then the legs kick out and the rib-cage comes together. The cycle of respiration matches the stride. Breath is the fuel for the muscles so the faster you go, the more breath you need.

A horse and rider from the Spanish Riding School of Vienna, in perfect harmony.

DANIEL PEVSNER
Dressage Instructor, Alexander Teacher, and student of the Spanish Riding School

I began taking Alexander lessons because my back was in pain whenever I got on to a horse, and because I was hoping to improve my riding position. The very first few lessons won me over completely. Everything was working well. The pain cleared, and I was changing shape quite dramatically. In time I found a great resemblance between the ideals of good posture and locomotion, as applied to horses or to people. The concepts and the procedures involved in attaining these ideals were not dissimilar. This to me was of the utmost importance. It dawned on me that, by learning this technique, I might achieve some of the equestrian experience that was then to me unobtainable. By studying the Technique, I was gaining a better understanding of horsemanship, and at the same time, my riding experience convinced me of the validity and the soundness of the Technique.

A further step in my development occurred some months later, when, in the autumn of '69, the Spanish Riding School of Vienna came to England. The school has been in existence for over 400 years and is today regarded as a custodian of the art of horsemanship. The kind of riding practiced in the school is called dressage. This can mean simply the basic schooling that every riding horse has to undergo, irrespective of what its job in life is going to be, but at its advanced level, dressage consists of high-school figures and movements, which, in equine locomotion, are the equivalent of human dance.

I had not seen the school perform live before, and the impact on me was quite staggering. The equestrian standard of the display was, of course, very high and very satisfying, but what struck me in particular were the superb use and posture of the riders. Although I was already at the time developing a new awareness and appreciation of good use, and even though by then I was a fairly experienced riding teacher, it was not until this meeting with the Spanish School that I realized to what extent one could develop one's own good use through correct riding. The riders before me were carrying themselves and acting as if they had all undergone thorough training in the technique. It then became obvious to me that in order to become a really top-class rider, one would have to develop qualities that would be instantly recognized and appreciated by an Alexander teacher.

RIDING A BICYCLE
JOE SEARBY

When you cycle and everything is going well, the upper body is fairly still, sitting bones contacting the saddle, spine lengthening, head going forward and up. The hands rest gently on the bars. You should be able to lift the hands off the bars without having to sit up much further. If the hands are resting lightly in this way, the elbows can remain free rather than braced and stiff or sticking out sideways. Contact can be made between the heel of the hand and the handlebars rather than just the fingers. This facilitates release of the hands/wrists onto the bars. An opening out of the shoulders is then encouraged. Handlebars should be wide enough to allow this. The pitched-forward position also puts pressure and strain on the shoulder joints, causing you to raise and round them.

With a better riding position, the lungs are allowed their full expansion and the spine is shock-absorbing. Roads are not always smooth, and shocks through the bike to the lumbar spine are a problem: most cyclists learn early to "lift" themselves out of the saddle over the bumps. Most cyclists are constantly trying to lift themselves out of the saddle anyway – like horse riders lifting themselves out of their seat. Most of the lower back pain suffered by cyclists is because of the riding position. The only part of the body that should really be moving is the legs. An upright position allows the legs to be used more independently of the torso, a bent-over position encourages the arms and torso to get involved. The bent-over posture

constricts the hips. The knees need to be brought forward rather than up or down and away from the ankles and hips. Hips back and down, calf back and down and out through the heel. The foot softens onto the pedal, to stop you from pushing with the foot. The ankle needs to be as free as possible. Think of the heel extending back and down to release over the front of the foot. The heels can extend out behind and the toes forward.

Design

The design of the modern bike has the rider's head low down and over the front wheel to cut to a minimum what he presents to the air. This has the effect of forcing the rider to lift his head to see where he is going and in most cases this is going to encourage a shortening at the back of the neck. This posture also causes excess bending at the lumbar spine and an extreme forward rotation of the pelvis/hips. This was and is considered advantageous because a bending of the spine in this way is thought to increase its shock-absorbing abilities! Classic racing advice was to have your saddle nose pointing up anyway. Racing cyclists may suffer temporary loss of fertility during their career. They also suffer from boils, piles, chafing, and sores.

One of the major advantages of making contact between the sitting bones and saddle is that you are better able to influence the direction of the bike through small shifts in body weight. In cycle racing you corner by leaning into the corner and using the leg as an extra weight, that is, you lean over and stick your knee out, as motorcyclists do in races. If the contact

Contact should be made between the heel of the hand and the handlebars.

When you sit correctly on the saddle, you have good control through small shifts of body weight.

NECK
SHORTENED

TENSION IN
WRISTS

Heading for a fall: the
rider has lost control of
himself and the bicycle.

When the weight is too far forward,
undue tension is created in the
elbows, shoulders, and wrists.

EXCESS PRESSURE
ON ANKLES

between seat and sitting bones is poor, this ability to move the bike without so much steering is diminished. This becomes important when you are going downhill at 60 mph/100 kph and oversteering could be fatal.

The obsession with the pitched-forward position persists. It has reached its extreme with modern "mountain bikes." In a competitive situation these bikes are ridden off the road, where speeds are too low for aerodynamics to make much difference, except in the case of "downhilling" where you go down an off-road hill as fast and directly as you can. The real problem comes when riders insist on using these bikes for ordinary road use. Everywhere you see riders straining their necks as they race down the high street to – the next set of traffic lights!

Despite all this doom and gloom, cyclists tend to suffer few injuries, except through accidents or collisions. Even ex-professionals tend to be relatively injury-free, apart from broken bones caused by collisions. The action of cycling is steady and rhythmic, even at high speeds, and a racing cyclist learns how to maintain a steady cadence (rate of pedal-stroke) by the use of the gears. Maintaining a regular pedal-stroke is fundamental to good racing, but is something generally

not understood by cyclists, especially mountain-bikers. By keeping your cadence (for racing cyclists this is something around 100–120 strokes/minute), you avoid large strains on the leg muscles, thus encouraging long muscle with a lot of stamina, rather than short muscle for bursts of activity. Using high gears at low speeds puts huge strains on the legs and very quickly tires them out. That is why bikes have gears and why professionals spend so much time learning how to use them properly. But you still see cyclists starting off from traffic lights in their higher gears, and you can bet that by the end of the trip their legs will hurt!

Constant repetition of the pedal-stroke can lead to problems in the long term. A tiny displacement of the foot will be magnified at the knee joint, and if the knee is then rotated thousands of times with that twist incorporated, you will certainly get knee problems. Cyclists seem generally unaware of this, yet many of them use shoes that clamp their foot to the pedal. These devices are useful in that they allow you to use the upstroke of the pedal as well as the downstroke, but the modern clamps require an outward twisting action of the foot that again can lead to knee problems. Better than these are "toe-straps" that go over the top of the foot and bind it to the pedal. The foot can be drawn straight out rather than twisted and the bindings can be left looser for quick release in case of accident. Racing cyclists tend to be completely clamped to the pedal, so if they fall they can't get their foot out. This total clamping reduces to a minimum the loss of energy from foot to pedal. The aim in racing is to convert as much of your energy as possible into forward motion. Therefore the frame and wheels are very stiff with little suspension. Modern mountain bikes now often have full suspension front and rear. This is useful if you are going downhill off-road, but on city streets it means your bike is absorbing half your motive energy. It's the difference between riding a bike made of steel and one made of rubber.

Cyclists also suffer from shortening of the hamstrings and of course the muscles of the legs. Most serious cyclists cannot touch their toes. They can also suffer tearing away of the tendons, hernias, and wrist damage (through too much weight being placed on the hands). Many people who cycle a lot and cycle hard are unaware of the damage they can cause themselves.

Damage Limitation Advice for Cyclists

- Don't come too far forward in the saddle
- Don't tighten your ankles
- Don't shorten the back of your neck
- Don't bend excessively at the lumbar spine
- Don't shorten the hamstrings
- Don't hold your breath in frantic bursts of pedaling

JOE SEARBY
Bicycle Designer and Alexander Technique Teacher

I learned to ride when I was 6 or 7, but I first started riding a bike every day when I was 11 as a means of getting to school and back. I was lucky enough to be brought up in Cambridge, England, where the bike is common and the hills are rare. After several years of at least six miles a day, I joined the local cycling club and began to train and race regularly. My love affair with training three nights a week and Sunday mornings and riding to school and back began to wane about the same time real love affairs appeared! However, I have never lost my love for bicycles and still ride every day.

Nearly everyone can ride a bike, and at one time in our lives we have all gained pleasure from freewheeling down a hill with the wind rushing past our ears. Cycling is almost a universal experience. It is both a very common solo and social activity and a sport. We all want that feeling of freedom and lightness, of effortless motion that freewheeling on a bike, sitting up with our hands off the handlebars, can give us. But so often we are head-down into the traffic fumes, hell-bent on getting somewhere. Even a lot of leisure cycling these days is competitive.

When all directions are going well, cycling is an effortless glide. It is possible to flow along with the muscles of the legs lengthening so that you can't feel the usual effort or tension. The hands on the bars encourage widening of the shoulders and an expansion of the ribcage. It feels as though you are being propelled by an outside energy rather than your own effort. That total combination of awareness and direction rarely lasts long (always another hazard to distract you), but while it does there's nothing like it. If you can manage to find a quiet road on a nice day, it can truly lift the heart and senses. That is cycling using the Technique. Without the Alexander Technique, cycling easily becomes a chore, a number of miles to do as fast as possible. Just as long as I beat that guy ahead of me ...

RUNNING
MALCOLM BALK

Good runners run tall, they do not hunch or lean. They run with the brakes off. There is an economy and integrity in their form and movement. They run smoothly. In many training circles today, coaches are emphasizing the importance of quality versus quantity work as the key to improvement and health. If a runner listens to the whispers, he won't have to listen to the screams. Many times a small niggle, if paid attention to, disappears, and enables a runner to survive and even thrive on the stresses imposed by high-quality training. The problem, if ignored, can turn into something more serious, as many runners and coaches will attest. Repeating something when you are injured or ill often leads to more of the same, or worse. Runners who pound often end up injured. Good runners run lightly – they don't try to dig holes in the ground with each stride. Alexander's belief is that if attention is paid to the means, the ends will take care of themselves. If this belief is taken into the world of training and racing, it allows the runner to take each day as it comes, to have confidence in the process, and enjoy it more.

The aim of the runner is to be fast, free, and light.

Running lightly has nothing to do with how much you weigh, but how light you feel.

Kenyan Runners

No wonder Kenyans are such good runners – look at their mothers. Kenyan women can be seen carrying heavy loads on their heads, with no loss of poise and, quite amazingly, no increase in their energy output. Yet they are able to walk for considerable distances over varied terrain without losing their equilibrium. This highlights the important role that head balance plays in movement. The head, no matter how great a runner you think you are, weighs about 10lbs/4.5kg.

The inherited natural poise and dynamic musculature gives Kenyans extraordinary stamina.

Advice for Runners

ALLOW YOUR ARMS to engage the legs through your back. Your shoulders need to remain free so the movement of the arms can connect with your legs through the back.

ALLOW YOUR ANKLES TO RELEASE. In order to allow your knees to bend freely, your ankles need to be free. Ask a friend to hold on to your ankle and try to bend your knee. You have to work hard to overcome the resistance. When they let go, your knee bends much more easily. Any holding in your ankles will make a smooth stride much less likely.

ALLOW YOUR KNEES, not your feet, to lead the movement forward. Trying to increase stride length by reaching forward with the foot results in a braking action and slows you down. It can cause you to lean back or sit on your hips rather than running tall.

ALLOW THE LEGS to move in a semicircular pattern. Good runners allow their legs to turn over in a semi-circular fashion with the heel approaching the buttock at the end of each stride, i.e. the knee bends at least 90 degrees before coming forward. Thinking of your legs moving in a circular rather than a linear way helps you develop a rhythmic running pattern, which is easier to maintain and modify according to your needs, for example, speeding up or running uphill.

ALLOW YOUR EYES to look 30–50 yards/30–50 meters ahead. When you look down, you often drop your head and neck as well. This makes you run heavily, as well as putting a strain on your neck and shoulders.

ALLOW THE EXTERNAL DIRECTION to be forward and the internal direction to be up. Many runners do not understand that although you may be moving forward in space, your spine does not have to go the same way. Ideally, as you are moving forward as a result of the action of your legs and feet, your spine with your head leading the way should be lengthening upward. This produces a lightness in your body, and as a result, your legs do not have to work so hard to move you forward.

LEARN TO RUN LIGHTLY AND QUIETLY. Pounding is a sign that something is wrong. Percy Cerutty suggested you run on the legs, not with the legs. You may be tired, not feeling well, or simply not paying attention. Running lightly has nothing to do with how much you weigh, as anyone with children who like to run around when you are trying to take a nap will attest. It has much more to do with attention – "listening to yourself as you run" – and intention, "thinking up." When runners pound, they literally jar their whole system. This can be blamed for much of the bad press that running has received in recent years.

ALLOW YOUR WRISTS TO REMAIN TONED, not floppy. Runners mistakenly run with their wrists so loose that their hands flop around. This belief that they are relaxed is actually creating unnecessary tension in the shoulders.

ALLOW YOUR ARMS to move forward and back in a straight line. This is the most effective arm movement for propelling you forward. A sprinter's upper arm will be parallel to the ground, both when it springs forward and when he pulls it back. The effort comes in pulling your arms back, not in pushing it forward. Pulling your arm back helps your legs pull you forward via your back.

ALLOW YOUR ELBOWS to remain bent at right angles. A short lever is more efficient since it requires less energy to move. Since you do want your arms to contribute to the running action, you need to know how this can be done as effectively as possible.

Keeping your head up and your eyes looking forward allows your whole body to lengthen upward.

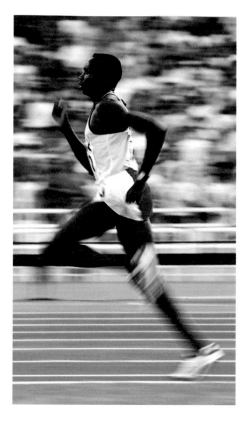

Wilson Kipketer's track success is based on a relaxed and efficient technique.

DON'T

- Push the body up and let it land heavily on the legs with every stride.
- Push with the feet.
- Lock the arms onto the trunk or fix the shoulders.
- Lock the feet to cross over the midline.
- Push (tuck) the pelvis into the legs – it is part of the back.
- Allow the head to roll, bob, or wag.
- Allow the fists to clench, the wrists to flop, the thumbs to stiffen.
- Clench the teeth and grimace.
- Bounce up and down or roll from side to side.
- Push the chest toward the target.
- Belly-breathe.

CASE STUDY

MALCOLM BALK
Runner and Alexander Technique Teacher

As a competitive athlete I had always run as part of playing baseball and football and once a year in the high-school track meet. In 1975 the running boom was in full swing. When my girlfriend declared her intention to run a marathon, I was stricken in more ways than one! Over the next five years I completed five marathons and managed to suffer a wide range of injuries common to many fellow marathoners: Achilles tendonitis, runner's knee, shin splints, calf, quad and hamstring pulls, etc … And although I managed to improve my times, there was a growing concern with a pattern that was becoming more apparent. As I put more and more time, effort, mileage, into running, I was getting less and less return. In 1981, I moved to England to begin training as a teacher of the Alexander Technique. I brought my cello with me and also kept up my running, now focusing on the 800. And it was here that the first effects of Alexander were being felt – literally. Although my training included several high sessions on the track familiar to every middle-distance runner, there was a big difference. I was no longer plagued with injuries in spite of maintaining a punishing level of high-quality training required for middle-distance running. Furthermore, up until my late 30s, my times kept getting faster, and now in my early 40s I maintain a level close to my personal bests. And still, NO INJURIES.

As he races, Malcolm Balk exhibits the good use necessary for success in the field.

SWIMMING
STEVEN SHAW

Swimming is generally regarded as one of the best forms of exercise, promoting a strong sense of health and well-being. The water takes the weight off the vertebrae, allowing for more release of the muscles. However, this is not always the case in practice, as the possibility of misuse is extremely high. Swimming with poor technique can actually do more harm than good. Bad style can aggravate old injuries and cause neck, shoulder, and back pain.

Water can be both frustrating and an extremely liberating medium to move through. When swimming, one finds oneself maneuvering within a substance that is a thousand times denser than air. As you push against it, it seems to do nothing but swirl away from you. On the other hand, the effects of buoyancy balancing the gravitational forces on the body open up a number of new and exciting possibilities for developing greater awareness and freedom of movement.

For a teacher of the Alexander Technique, it is particularly relevant to look at the head-neck-back relationship in swimming. In the buoyant environment of a swimming pool, even small changes in this relationship can have a very considerable effect on the functioning of the body. The common tendency of

NATURAL
BUOYANCY

holding the head out of the water while swimming on the front can produce a significant strain on the whole of the back, which reduces the efficiency of movement. In contrast, releasing the neck so the head rests in the water helps to free the rest of the body, allowing the swimmer to float higher and move with greater ease. Thus, one of the first obstacles to be overcome is the reluctance to place one's face in the water. As a teacher one frequently observes swimmers with their heads held clear of the water who swim relatively fast, but who are thrown into panic when water splashes unexpectedly in their face. Many people often have a false notion that if they submerge their face, they will inevitably breathe in water. Learning to overcome this fear through the application of inhibition is a vital first step. There is little point swimming up and down a pool if you are not completely at ease in water.

The water offers the opportunity to breathe in a much freer way. The physical support provided by the water reduces the requirement for oxygen. Clinical trials have discovered a "diving instinct" that is present in most mammals including human beings; exhaling with the whole face submerged results in a slow-down of the metabolic rate. Tests show significant reductions in both cardiovascular activity and levels of blood pressure. Few swimmers take advantage of these phenomena. While

The Alexander Technique allows swimmers to find their true length while in the water.

BODY SUPPORTED
BY WATER

LENGTHENED
BACK

The head should not be held out of the water since it can produce a strain on the whole of the back.

in the water most people are more likely to disturb and interfere with their natural breathing process than they would be outside of the water. This can be attributed partly to the effects of anxiety and partly to an overestimation of the amount of air required to move through the water. People suck in large quantities of air, as if they were about to swim a whole length underwater. If too much air is inhaled, there isn't enough time to exhale it all before the next point of inhalation. This is the major cause of breathlessness and hyperventilation. In both the crawl and the breaststroke, inhalation ought to be smooth and gentle. Breathing should be focused on the exhalation with the face remaining in the water until all the air is expelled. Then, simply raising the head and opening the mouth allows a natural breathing pattern to provide enough oxygen to continue. Holding the breath underwater confuses and disturbs both the natural breathing mechanism and the rhythm of the stroke.

Stand holding the rail and exhale into the water, first submerging the mouth only, then the mouth and nose, then, finally, the whole of the face. When you feel comfortable and relaxed with the whole of the face under the water, you may let go of the bar and move onto gliding. Obviously, the amount of time it takes individual students to overcome this difficulty varies tremendously. However, I have yet to meet anyone who, with the right teaching support, has not been able to overcome this fear.

CASE STUDY

STEVEN SHAW
Author of **The Art of Swimming**

While training to become an Alexander teacher, I worked at a health spa as a lifeguard and swimming instructor. The pool was seldom very busy, which gave me plenty of opportunity to experiment in the water. Being a competitive swimmer, I always considered myself as having good style. However, through my lessons in the Alexander Technique I began to notice that I was misusing myself quite badly.

Probably the deepest problem I faced concerned my approach to swimming. After years of plowing up and down the pool aiming to increase my speed, I found it difficult to get into the water without working to a set of preset goals such as completing a certain number of lengths in a given time. I realized that my relationship to swimming was one of an extreme end-gainer. As I started to control this tendency, I began to discover that the water offered me a wonderful opportunity to free myself, and for the first time since I was a young child I actually began to enjoy being in the water. When I recently attended a reunion of my swimming team, it was interesting to note that most of them no longer swam and said that they did not enjoy swimming any more.

When I began teaching swimming, I found that the tendency toward end-gaining was also a major obstacle for noncompetitive swimmers. Many swim in order to get fitter, strengthen their muscles, or lose weight, and as a result they have set ideas about what they should do to achieve these aims. Little thought is given to the way they move through the water, and automatic habits take over. Therefore it is vital that students reconsider their motivation for being in the water before they can move toward developing a new way of swimming. It is very important when learning to improve swimming skills that students do not limit themselves by trying to do it the "right way." What is required is a much more experimental approach. Unfortunately, pools are public places where people feel self-conscious, which is part of the reason that swimmers seem unwilling to experiment in the water. This contrasts with the sense of security achieved in the private domain of an Alexander teaching room. Feelings of self-consciousness must be overcome in order to develop a new understanding and way of being in water.

TENNIS
JACK MACDONALD

You cannot be serious!

How many times has a game of tennis gone from being a lovely invitation to play in the warm sun, with strawberries for tea, to a frenzy of racket throwing and total disappointment in yourself, the game, and the day? But what is required to avoid this? Concentration is really the major factor in tennis, not just on the score, or whether to play a lob or a volley, but concentration on how you are working yourself. Are you breathing properly? Where is your strength coming from? Are you finding that you stamp across the court while others seem so graceful?

There are times when you have a minute to pause, balance yourself, and then continue with the game. At these points, find the breath again, focus on the space around you, and strive for the key word – fluidity. Often people play whole games of tennis with the words "game, set, match" galloping around their minds and rarely concentrate on each stroke they play. This method of playing an "end" rather than a "game" generally causes us to tense up, which in turn causes us to speed up, which in turn causes us to give up.

Take your time. Free your neck. Keep your balance. Put your back into it.

The Serve

1. You are at the baseline. If you raise the toes of your front foot, this will guide your weight onto your back foot. At this point, focus on where you want to place the ball and how you are going to do it. Think and breathe out.

2. If you think of the direction above your head as 12 o'clock, it is best to throw the ball above you to about 2 o'clock. This enables you to put your full weight behind you as you jump into the serve. Stretch and lengthen. Your eyes should be firmly fixed on the ball from now until contact. Follow the ball with your throwing arm as if reaching for it and at the same time turn your hips as a unit.

3. So the racket is raised ready for contact with the ball. Your weight should shift onto your forward foot as you make contact. As you keep your body connected, you will be poised for a powerful serve.

4. Try to keep your neck free and your back lengthened and widened. Do not brace your legs or stiffen your ankles. As your throwing arm is dropped, you should simultaneously drop the racket down your back. Now launch toward the moment of contact, while rotating your front hip. Stretch is the buzz-word as you use your full size and weight to make contact with the ball.

5. Try to land within the court. Your head should remain up, enabling you to move quickly toward the net if necessary – play the game.

CASE STUDY

JACK MacDONALD
Tennis Player

I began playing tennis when I was 8 years old and found that I had problems in three areas. First, I was growing very fast – I had big feet, big hands, and a long back, but was very skinny. Second, I had a terrible tendency to give up if the going got tough or if I felt I couldn't win. I felt I had no choice but to be the champion. By not end-gaining or worrying so much about the outcome of the match before I had played a stroke, I began to be able to keep going and not give up. This in turn steadied my nerves, and I did not care so much if I lost a point but just kept playing. Third, I had no control over my breath. This was partly due to being so keen to win I forgot to breathe and also I forgot to have fun, so there was very little laughter on the court. Through stopping and directing, my breathing pattern got easier. By doing whispered "Ah's" I had more breath, and sometimes the thought of something funny released into a laugh which helped enormously. I had more energy and found I could play a five-set match, and even tie-breaks became easier. The Alexander Technique helped me in all these areas and enabled me to give my directions, be aware of lengthening and widening, and use my joints so I knew where my arms and legs started and stopped. This gave me a greater confidence as I realized my space, my posture came together, and my strokes became easier. I feel I can control my height and use it to its full. The real benefit came with the development that occurred in the control over my breath. Suddenly my brain and blood were receiving vital oxygen, and my game really picked up.

Helpful Tennis Tips

STOP

1. Use your eyes and expand your vision.
2. Give your directions and come up to your full height.
3. Find your fluidity.
4. Picture the shot you want.
5. Breathe out and find your internal space and your space on court.

NEVER
GIVE UP

GOLF
GORDON MCCAFFREY

At the time of my first Alexander lesson I had been, for at least ten years, the stereotypical golf fanatic, and my original motivation for the lessons was as an aid to golf improvement. For anyone similarly inclined it may be of interest to read how, through practice of the Technique, golf was transformed for me from an addictive drudgery to an enjoyable sport.

For at one time I was so keen to improve and discover the secret of golf that I practiced three times weekly and in one frenzied year played and practiced every single day. In looking for this key to perfect golf I supplemented this practice with a comprehensive reading program of golf instructional literature. All the advice of the great players and teachers was analyzed in theory, then attempted on the course; all to no avail. I was left wandering in the literary labyrinth of contradictory instruction where the path of "use all hands" tempted me from the way of "no hands all body," and the direction of good posture was pointed out by guides with clearly distorted spines. It was from this maze that by great luck I stumbled out into the light provided by the Alexander Technique.

CASE STUDY

GORDON MCCAFFREY
Alexander Teacher and Amateur Golfer

It was around 15 years ago I started having lessons in the Alexander Technique and quickly discovered that what the experience did for me overall was much more important than my narrow golfing objective. Over the years, as my general use improved, I started to discard golf theory and just swing through the ball while maintaining a better use of myself. It was this practical procedure, called the Alexander Technique, which enabled me to swing through the ball with better use.

In the first six months of lessons, a whole new world of self-observation was opened up to me. Until then I had never given any thought to what I did to myself as I sat in a chair, bent to pick up a book, washed the dishes, etc. My teacher was able to make me aware that my preparation for these acts was wrong and inappropriate. Gradually I began to see clearly that this wrong preparation was present when I played golf, even when I took my clubs out of the locker, teed up my ball, took my grip, or assessed and planned my next shot. So as I gained experience in the prevention of the wrong habitual preparation in my everyday activities, I realized that my golf game was nothing more than a continuation of these activities and not something separate.

From then on, my interest in my general use became much more important to me than my previously introverted obsession with golf mechanics.

Amazingly, to me at least, I found that when practicing less and less, I could still play to my low single-figure handicap. Now, after teaching the Alexander Technique for over ten years, I am certain that my experience with golf, this elimination of practice and absorption with golf methods while still playing well, would equally apply to other sports and activities. Of course, the conclusion must not be drawn that an interest in practicing or technique is harmful. It is the use of the self while implementing the instruction or even reading the advice which is all-important. It will soon dawn on any golfer who takes Alexander lessons, as I did, that he or she is involved in something more comprehensive than a golf game.

As my general use improved, so did my golf game, but so also to a far greater extent did my enjoyment of the sport, of being on the course, the stimulation of looking and seeing all around me. This corresponded to a reduction in false concentration causing tension and exhaustion. To be able to enjoy the drive to the course, the game, the company, the drive home, and the rest of the day is such a happy contrast to my early years in golf. For me, my search for "the secret" was a success, but a far greater secret was revealed along the way.

SKIING
VIVIEN GREEN

When you first put on your skis, walk around on the flat. Having a different weight and length on your feet because of your boots and skis completely alters your balance. It is helpful to get used to this change before you go onto the slope.

Check that your hips are directly underneath your shoulders and that you are standing in a balanced way, with the weight equally distributed on both feet. Think of the cross-pattern connections – that is, your right hip connecting to your left shoulder and your left hip connecting to your right shoulder as you line up. This will help you to not shorten and contract as you find the body pattern that you need.

Think of widening through your upper back and let your arms hang loosely by your sides. Check that you are not gripping your ski poles.

Gently nod your head forward, and as you do breathe out and let your weight follow the direction of your head. As your weight transfers and moves forward, you can turn the skis and off you go. The conscious

Let your knees bend forward so you are leaning onto the front of your ski boots. This is a good moment to check again that you are not overpreparing for your descent by stiffening. Breathe out again.

Bend your elbows and hold the poles slightly off the ground. Breathe out again to help release any tension in your shoulders and upper back.

CASE STUDY

VIVIEN GREEN
Natural Health Consultant

I first started the Alexander Technique when I was pregnant. I used to go along with a huge bump of a baby and after the lesson, because my back had lengthened and widened, there was more space for the baby to move back and the bump had almost disappeared! I decided to try and apply the principles of the Alexander Technique the next time I went skiing. I remember putting on my skis and thinking, keep the neck free, breathe out, lengthen the spine, connect the lower back muscles, release as I bend my knees. My skiing improved vastly. I floated down the slope, all the time gently reminding myself to smile and breathe out, and the difference was remarkable. When I came to a difficult area, I found myself tensing and losing the fluidity, but with the simple reminder of breathing out and releasing the whole situation changed.

As with all sports, accidents occur when the fear reflex is activated. The body tenses, and falls become far more serious. So always watch young children and learn to keep their sense of fun and fearlessness so when things go awry the rubber ball reflex can be activated, laughter comes to the surface, and the tension can be released to make falling an easy art. By the way, never look at adults beginning if you are a beginner – not good examples!

awareness that the Alexander Technique teaches you is very important for skiing. This awareness is particularly important when you consider your joints, especially the knee joint and how easily it can be damaged. Because the ankle is immobilized by the boots, greater pressure is exerted on this joint. So getting it well exercised before you go off on the slopes is important. Practice bending and squatting to strengthen your knees and keep them mobile.

WORKING OUT

I see
The lost are like this and their scourge to be
As I am mine, their sweating selves; but worse.

GERARD MANLEY HOPKINS: *CARRION COMFORT*

In order to get the most out of your work in the gym and make sure that you do not injure yourself, you must begin by warming up properly. Not only does a proper warmup ease out your muscles and get them working, it helps to put you in the right frame of mind for exercise. If your mental attitude is incorrect, you may approach your exercise in an unfocused way, rushing or using too much weight in your enthusiasm to achieve results *(see End-gaining, page 35)*. As in every activity, how you do what you do determines a successful outcome.

Often people make the mistake of stretching in a jerky fashion, or they exert excessive muscular effort to pull themselves into a stretch. This can lead to injury. Instead, let your body weight ease you into the stretch. If you listen to your muscles, they will tell you when you have reached the point of tension. Stop stretching at this moment and just rest there. Allow your neck to be free so your head can release on the atlanto-occipital joint, drop your shoulders and allow the weight of your arms to help you increase the space

BAD USE IS
POTENTIALLY
DAMAGING

through your upper chest. You will find that when you release the resistance in your body, your body weight is then able to do your stretching for you and exert the appropriate "pull" on the muscles.

Rowing Machine

The Rowing Machine is a useful place to apply the Alexander Technique in the gym.

The question of how much effort you should be expending is important, and in the end it is a personal matter. But no matter what your aims are, when using resistance equipment, it is important that you exercise with care and intelligence. If you pull yourself out of shape or generate inappropriate tension in the process, then your results will reflect this. If you avoid tightening in the head–neck–back area, you will sense that you are sitting on a mechanism that glides back and forth, and it will help you to judge when you start to make counter-productive effort. Remember that you are trying to develop strength and not shortened muscles that leave the body distorted, out of shape, and muscle bound. So it is important that you register when you start to shorten your stature as you increase muscular energy.

As you start, work with the least resistance possible. This allows you to build up gradually. As you add more resistance, you can be aware of the feedback from your whole body, particularly the head, neck, and upper back, and not just the effort that you are exerting. When you come forward in the machine, it is important that you don't come down in front and restrict the breathing.

DO NOT STIFFEN
YOUR NECK. DO
NOT HOLD YOUR
BREATH

The rowing machine is an excellent piece of resistance equipment that is of great help to the cardiovascular system if used correctly.

Exercise Bike

It is not uncommon when riding the exercise bike machine for people to use inappropriate effort by pulling their heads back, raising their shoulders, and shortening the front of the body. What they fail to realize is that not only are they distorting the body's framework, but they are failing to exercise the intended muscles.

When you have taken hold of the handles, pause before you start pedaling. Release your neck and let the weight take your arms up and out from your back. Relax up the front of your body. Now let the hips drop down and be aware of the back running up from the pelvis and fanning out into your shoulders and arms. Instead of using just the legs to pedal, think that the legs are an extension of the whole body and that when you lengthen into the action, this allows the whole of your back to share the work.

As you release your muscles and let the legs return to their resting place, allow the air to come in through your nose. Pause for a moment and release the muscles of your neck, back, shoulders, and arms so the full length of the back from the base of your sitting bones to your hands can be restored. Then start pedaling again.

As you get tired, bored, or overenthusiastic, you may pull your body down. This is an indication that you have reached your limit. It is important you stop the exercise and recover your full height and the integrity of your body before you continue.

LET YOUR
HEAD GO
FORWARD
AND UP

MAINTAIN YOUR
FULL HEIGHT

Exercise Hints

Why do we exercise? To get fit. Fit for what? Fit for life. How to get the best out of exercise and maximize the beneficial effects:

TAKE TIME. Devote some undisturbed period of time to every thing you do and prepare yourself and your environment so you can be undisturbed while exercising – turn off the mobile phone.

BE COMFORTABLE – work in good positions only – do not go for the burn.

PERSIST – repetition multiplies effect.

CONNECT – keep reminding yourself of its effect on everyday activities.

WORK IN SILENCE – talk dissipates energy.

DUMBBELLS

Preparation

The Alexander Technique is not the main transforming agent; your desire for change is the motivator. Senseless, aggressive energy causes pain. This energy can be directed against yourself, and after a time this intense energy of aggression leads to psychological ills.

There is a growing number of people who train as hard as professional sportsmen. They train for and compete in incredible feats of endurance while also holding down jobs or careers. What they don't have is the backup of physios, trainers, the very best doctors and surgeons! What they forget is that professional sports people suffer a lot of injury; it's just that they expect it and are prepared for it. Ordinary people don't have that backup, yet they insist on doing things that will damage them. Then when they do get damaged, their only concern is how quickly can they be fixed, manipulated, or operated on to sort it out so they can get back to competing! The idea of simply enjoying sport is being forgotten. These days it's all about faster times, greater distances, more punishment of the self!

The exercise bike is a useful way of building up your stamina

GARDENING

Alexander compared his Technique to gardening, believing that there were no satisfactory shortcuts in either. Gardening, which gives us such pleasure, is also demanding work. Such is our enthusiasm to create our little Eden that we often work for longer and more energetically than is good for us. We get out in April, having not had much exercise over the winter months, and work like mad, and end up putting a fork through our toes or pruning the wrong branch. At the end of the day we are stiff and tired and even injured, with aching muscles, sprained joints, and stretched ligaments. More haste, less speed.

Standing

If we start at ground level, preparing the soil is one of the first jobs we have to do. When using shovels, forks, and rakes, we need to stand in the upright position. How you take hold of the tool you are using is very important. Quite often, we put too much effort into gripping the handle. See how lightly you can hold the tool without letting it slip from your grasp. So as you begin to rake, dig, and hoe, the amount of energy required will increase, but this does not mean you have to overtighten your grasp. Your long back muscles can do more of the work. Remember to keep your neck free and your head going forward and up as you perform each movement.

This principle applies especially when you are digging; it is not necessary to put huge amounts of energy into the action. You do not have to push quite so hard when you remember that the shovel is designed to cut through the soil. When it is laden with soil, remember to counterbalance the heavy weight your arms are carrying by coming back, onto your heels. If you maintain the two-way stretch in your back you will have more elasticity in your muscles to cope with lifting.

Good advice for gardeners is to take frequent breaks and vary your chores – do not remain too long in any job. When you have done some digging, change to a task that allows you to sit or kneel or stretch upward.

Sitting and Kneeling

Many jobs in the yard are done in the kneeling position. Edging, weeding, planting in small holes, and sowing all take a lot of time – it is no bad thing to be slowed down. The knee joint is not really designed to bear a lot of weight for any length of time. When kneeling is the appropriate position to be in for your task, use a garden mat to help reduce pressure on your knee joints. When you move, crawling on all-fours is an excellent way to move from place to place as you can give your back a rest, allowing it to release and lengthen out in opposite directions (see Crawling, page 80). Again, do not grasp the clippers or trowel too tightly, and take frequent breaks between jobs.

Remember to get into a stable position before doing repetitive work.

Remember to keep your neck free and let your head going forward as you dig.

Do not stiffen your neck when you pick up awkward bundles.

Don't forget to take frequent breaks.

Bending and Lifting

These actions, moving up and down, are an essential part of gardening, but are the most common cause of injuries, often serious. Sacks of soil, bags of refuse, even armfuls of dead leaves need to be moved, but you should be thoughtful about "how" you go about these tasks. When you get the bags out of the car, try the principles of the position of mechanical advantage.

If you feel you have strained your back lifting or carrying, take a few moments to lie in the semi-supine position *(see page 78)* and allow gravity to help your body return to a released position. Why not look up at the sky and plan what to do next in the yard? Take time to stop and enjoy what your labors are producing.

Nothing is so beautiful as Spring –
When weeds, in wheels, shoot long
and lovely and lush;
Thrush's eggs look little low heavens ...

GERARD MANLEY HOPKINS: SPRING

Pushing and Stretching Up

Pushing a mower or wheelbarrow demands a lot of back muscle work. When you free your neck and allow your back to lengthen and widen, the whole body shares the workload. The dangerous action is often the pulling back of the mower, rather than pushing it. Remember, as in all activities, to breathe out. By holding your breath, you will be creating unnecessary pressure in the chest and not getting enough oxygen.

When you need to stretch up, remember that you can look up quite freely, but you need to be conscious of how you let your head bend backward. Often the cutters are very unwieldy, and you can tend to overtense when holding them up to try to reach the high branches. Lower branches that need holding with one hand and cutting with the other can tend to narrow in the upper chest and back. Try not to clutch the tools too tightly.

Remember to breathe out when exerting yourself.

Do not overtighten when maneuvering heavy loads. Remember to always stay balanced.

Keep your neck free when you look up.

BUILDING AND DECORATING

These days, many of us decide to decorate our own homes. Do it yourself – the very phrase makes us feel responsible – we do not need the expert, we can do it ourselves. This puts a real responsibility on us. How do we know we can do it? You had better check out "yourself" before assuming you can "do it."

Everyone who has tried to do a job for himself has at some stage blamed the tools – that wretched screwdriver, that hopeless paintbrush that left hairs on every stroke, that useless drill that could not make an impression on the wall. "I'll replace that – it's not worth another moment's grief."

Perhaps we are the problem, not the tools. "A bad workman always blames his tools." Are we bad workmen? And is that "badness" no more than being unconscious

USE THE
RIGHT TOOLS

of the fact that we are to blame, not the tools? We are the first tool that needs to be checked, long before we abuse the screwdriver or drill or saw.

When you come to painting large surfaces, the usual brush is often replaced by the roller, which spreads a significantly greater area with paint. The danger is that the very nature of a large area full of potentially dripping paint makes the roller quite a tool with which to reckon. The Alexander Technique helps with painting by reminding you to pause before any action.

In the case of roller painting, this is essential, otherwise, you end up with an overfilled roller, the need to get it onto the wall and the real fear that it will drip everywhere. These are all stimuli to make you overtighten and hold your breath, which can lead to stiffness in your shoulders and neck.

Do not overtense your wrist and hand when holding a brush. The handle follows the line of your arm.

USE BACK MUSCLES

When you need to apply pressure, use your strong back muscles not just the muscles of the forearm.

CASE STUDY

ROGER KIDD
Alexander Teacher

The Nature of the Work – Floor tiling is a very physical craft. It involves a lot of lifting and carrying heavy tiles and bags of cement, bending down, kneeling for long periods while reaching and twisting. All these actions have to be carried out carefully with attention to detail, because the end result has to look good.

The Problem – I was getting aches and stiffness in my lower back and knees. As the jobs had to be done in a reasonable time (both for myself and the client), I would then throw myself into the work with more hurried brute strength. This approach not only made the stiffness worse, but also made me clumsier, forcing me to spend even more time in these awkward positions correcting my mistakes.

The Solution – The Alexander Technique showed me how I was tensing up well before the point when I could usually feel it (after a long period of kneeling). This then enabled me to avoid these unnecessary tensions before setting about the work, so I could see how I could lift and carry heavy bags of cement without bracing and holding my breath; bend down repeatedly without effort; reach and turn while kneeling without any strain and stiffness. All this let me work more easily and more quickly without the hurry. I am more efficient in my work, and I have more energy because I am no longer wasting it.

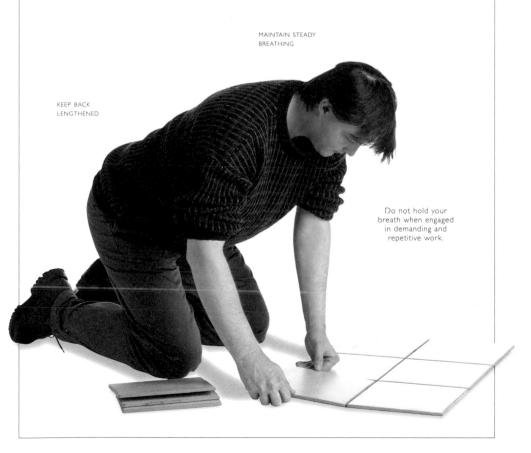

MAINTAIN STEADY
BREATHING

KEEP BACK
LENGTHENED

Do not hold your
breath when engaged
in demanding and
repetitive work.

HOUSEHOLD CHORES

We have all benefited from the skills of the designer in our homes. Our kitchens are time-and-motion studies that aim to conserve our energy by reducing how far we have to walk between appliances, by making the height of the work surfaces appropriate, and by generally styling the work surfaces and door handles to be ergonomically correct. Yet despite all these practical advantages, we still manage to spill hot dishes, cut our fingers, slip and fall, and burn the food.

A little more study of our own time and motion would pay off. We rush from job to job, without paying due attention to how we are performing. We are always making lists of jobs to be done, from a list of ingredients, to shopping, to the menus, to the order of preparation. What would it be like if we made a few notes for ourselves?

If we had this memo board, we could refer to it as we went from job to job. By taking the time to prepare ourselves before the action, we would be less likely to injure ourselves. Let us look at the familiar job of chopping vegetables.

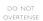

DO NOT
OVERTENSE

Chopping

Think of how you are standing before you begin. Do not stiffen your knees or lock your ankles, but allow your knees to flex gently and your hip bones to move slightly back, so you are beginning to bend. When you pick up the knife, try not to grasp it too tightly, and do not hold your breath. When you begin to chop, try not to hunch your shoulders, and try to have your knife sharp, so you do not have to put too much effort into pressing down on the handle. When you have chopped for a while, stop and take a break. Move from this position and do some other job for a moment, so your muscles do not lock into the repetitive chopping mode. Taking these momentary breaks will not waste your time, but allow you to resume your task efficiently and probably do it faster and better.

So often energy is wasted by putting too much effort into simple jobs. Next time you are taking the lid off a jar, check how much you are gripping the jar, and see whether you can unscrew it with half the effort. The same principles apply to any job done in the kitchen,

especially washing dishes. Remember to keep your mind on the job that you have at hand and do not fall into the trap of end-gaining (seeing it finished) or thinking of something else altogether. Each action is complete in itself, so the cup or plate you are washing at this very moment is the only thing that you are thinking about. Thinking about something else to take your mind off what you are doing, because you do not enjoy it, is a pointless exercise. Paying attention to the job at hand makes it interesting.

Lifting and Carrying

Another area that can cause problems is the lifting and carrying of heavy pots and dishes, often full of hot food. The expectation that something is going to be heavy to lift often makes us stiffen (see Lifting, page 75). When you add to this the fear of possibly getting burned, or dropping a carefully and expensively prepared dish on the floor, the excitation of the fear reflex increases and we overtighten.

The way you prepare to lift is very important. Take a moment to free your neck and give your

DO NOT STIFFEN
YOUR WRISTS

directions, then test the weight of the dish or pot and whether your gloves or oven mitts really protect you from the heat source. So often you only realize that the gloves are not working when you are half-way across the kitchen. Being conscious of how you perform these actions will decrease the likelihood of straining or burning yourself.

Ironing

The way you stand at the ironing board and the very way you get the board set up are important.

Do not grip the iron tightly, nor press down too heavily. If you apply the principles of Inhibition and Direction, you will achieve a good result without aching shoulders and back.

MAINTAIN YOUR
FULL HEIGHT

Vacuuming

Vacuuming is one of the most common sources of back injury in the home. Suddenly, for no apparent reason, our back suddenly gives out. We are bent double over the vacuum cleaner, unable to straighten up or to bend to switch off the power. Why does this happen? One explanation is that we are pushing and pulling a relatively heavy object back and forth, and not paying enough attention to the way we are using our bodies to counterbalance the weight of the appliance. As we continue with the activity, we are lulled into an almost semiconscious state by the repetitive nature of the physical movement and the numbing sound of the appliance. We are expending physical energy in an almost robotic state. Our muscles decide this is not wise;

Be careful when vacuuming that you let your body weight move forward and back as a counterbalance to the appliance.

USE YOUR WEIGHT AS A COUNTER BALANCE

DO NOT HOLD YOUR BREATH

DO NOT PULL DOWN IN FRONT

using too much activity with no thought for how the primary control is working makes them rebel and go into spasm.

How do you stay conscious in a repetitive task? If you keep thinking of your directions and get a good breathing rhythm established, you can avoid the robotic state that can induce muscular reaction that ends in pain or even injury. By waking up the conscious response, even the most seemingly mundane task can be satisfactorily performed.

Sewing

The first thing to do when you want to sew or knit is to consider how you sit. To begin, your weight should be on your sitting bones and your feet on the floor. Your body should not be leaning forward putting weight on the thighs and causing the muscles of the legs and abdomen to lighten. When you pick up your work, you should compensate for the weight of your arms and work by allowing the torso to lean slightly backward in the same way as a musician has to counterbalance the weight

of his instrument. You can lean back against a supporting pillow.

The great temptation as you get engrossed in your work is to allow your eyes to draw you nearer and nearer to your work so you end up with the work in your lap and your back a semi-circle.

So support yourself comfortably on a firm pillow, raise your arms toward your eyes, and enjoy your creativity. Whatever one is doing, the important thing is to remain in balance.

I have always found sewing a great test of the principles of the Alexander Technique.
DILYS CARRINGTON

MASSAGE
ANNA PALLANT

Massage, like the Alexander Technique, involves hands-on contact with people. The massage therapist must be constantly aware of the "connectedness of the body" and the integrity of the spine. She must also be able to stop her own tendencies to try too hard to help her patient. Naturally, the aim is to help the person, but by trying too hard the massage therapist can cause unnecessary tension in herself, especially in her shoulders and hands.

If a massage therapist has taken Alexander Technique lessons, her own posture will be comfortable, and she will be able to work with freedom and clarity. Her hands will be light and strong. The direction in which the muscles need to move in order to release will be clearly indicated.

When patients having massage therapy have previously had lessons in the Alexander Technique, they seem to respond very quickly and receive maximum benefits in terms of balance, relaxation, and well-being.

Practical

Working in a position of mechanical advantage is essential when massaging. Massage therapists are standing for most of the day using their arms and hands on their patients. Often their legs can get tired, causing referred pain in the lower back. Applying the principles of the Alexander Technique by remembering to stop and free the neck, to let the head go in a forward-and-up direction, often reduces this tiredness and pain.

HEALING HANDS

The poise, strength, and lightness of the massage therapist will be transmitted to the patient.

DO'S

- Breathe out while applying pressure through the hands.
- Bend in a good way by remembering the position of mechanical advantage.
- Widen through the upper back and shoulders.
- Think of the shoulders, elbows, and wrists as tunnels.

DONT'S

- Hold the breath.
- Stiffen the wrists.
- Tighten and narrow in the shoulders.
- Try too hard to help.

CASE STUDY

ANNA PALLANT,
Artist and Aromatherapist

I have found the Alexander Technique very helpful in my work as an aromatherapist massage practitioner. I started taking Alexander Technique lessons at about the same time as I began my aromatherapy training. At this time I was having frequent headaches and my posture was poor.

Through the Alexander Technique work I learned how my body tenses up, and I learned how to stop and then to direct myself out of these old patterns of use that were causing my problems.

When I see someone in need, I want to be of help to them; but if I try too hard and make too much effort, I often defeat my desired end by becoming tense myself and less effective. So often the more one does, the less productive the massage becomes. It seems the massage is most effective when I am equally conscious of both myself as the massage practitioner and my patient. Then I can be present without being intrusive. Each time I move a limb or work on releasing the spine, I am aware of how their whole system connects up.

One question which my clients often ask at the end of their massage is, "What can I do for myself to help prevent tension, painful back, headache, stiff neck?" My answer would be to have a course of Alexander Technique lessons. It worked for me.

DRIVING A CAR
JOE SEARBY

Loughborough University researchers in England have shown that people who spend more than half their working day driving, or drive over 25,000 miles a year, are more likely to suffer from lower back problems that cause absence from work. They are also three times more likely than average to suffer from disk problems.

It is easy to suffer from driving because it is such a demanding task. You are in charge of a potentially lethal instrument surrounded by other lethal weapons, so underlying anxiety levels must be high. You are squashed into a seat that has little to do with the human body, and you have to use both arms and legs almost continually, while remaining alert and focused.

Most of the problems suffered by drivers (apart from accidents) come from being in a fixed position or posture for long periods while being vibrated and bounced around and hanging onto the steering wheel. People drive themselves into the ground.

Car seats pose particular problems. The seat slopes backward and in any car more than a few years old is usually too soft and collapsed. It will invariably be more collapsed on one side, usually the right. Many cars offer lumbar supports (adjustable), but these are generally more of a curse than a blessing. Because they push the lumbar spine forward, they prevent it from flattening and weaken the supporting muscles, so exacerbating any present condition. Better is a firm seat wedge that gives more support and encourages a better use of the lower back, allowing it to be mobile and strengthening the postural muscles (provided general use is good). However, if you are over five feet five inches, unless you drive a convertible or a big truck, you are unlikely

Remember to turn the head freely when looking in the rearview mirror.

to have the headroom to be able to use a wedge. You could try a triangular-shaped wedge in the corner of the seat where it meets the back, or a piece of wood on the seat is also recommended. People also tend to have the seat back too reclined, so the upper back gets no support at all as they pull themselves forward toward the wheel. Then they have to pull their head back to look forward. Their elbows are rigid, shoulders hunched, head to one side, hands gripping the wheel. Holding the foot over the clutch leads to tension in the whole leg. Allowing the accelerator foot to fall to one side on long journeys can lead to problems in the knee or ankle.

The angle between the torso and legs is never going to be ideal (always too acute), but you can minimize discomfort by making sure you don't have to stretch for the pedals, also that you are not scrunched up into the steering wheel. Cars are all made for people of average height, so it is bad luck if you're not.

Sit well back in the seat, making good contact with the whole of your back.

Let the head turn the whole upper body when you look around.

Before you Drive

Take a moment before you get in to the car to stop and stand still. Allow your feet to soften onto the ground. Allow your head to go up to your full height. Let your shoulders release down, away from your ears. Don't become caught up in thinking about getting to your destination. Think about the process of driving – about how you are going to get there, not when.

Remember that your state of mind before you set off will be translated into your driving, so if you are anxious or angry or in a rush, take a short time to release these negative emotions. Bring your awareness to your own breathing and allow it to be gentle and easy. Allow the out-breath to carry away any negativity and tension. Avoid anything that has an effect on the central nervous system and increases stress, such as lots of coffee or cigarettes. Get into the car slowly and easily instead of throwing in your briefcase and then yourself after it!

Take your time and breathe out before you set off.

Stand with your back to the car seat with both feet on the ground. Ease yourself onto the seat and swing both feet into the car. Remember that driving is not automatic – it requires awareness and concentration.

Sitting Position

Sit well back in the seat so that the mid- to upper back makes contact with the back of the seat, especially between the shoulder blades. Don't lean your head back on the headrest. Keep your face going forward. Have the back of the seat about 10 degrees behind the vertical so that you are leaning back slightly. Make sure you are not stretching to reach the pedals, but that you are not scrunched up against the steering wheel either. Have your hands at the classic ten-to-two on the wheel with the elbows bent so the arms aren't stretched. Don't grip the wheel too strongly. Allow the wrists rather than the fingers to make the stronger contact with the wheel. Feel that the arms are providing support through the mid-back, making you four-footed. Allow your weight down into the seat while allowing your head to go up "through the roof." The use of a solid foam seat wedge can be very beneficial. This is a thinnish wedge that is angled down toward the front of the seat.

Do not stretch to reach the pedals.   Do not lounge in the driving seat.   Do not peer through the windshield

During the Drive

Make sure your left foot does not hover over the clutch, but is resting flat on the floor when not in use. When waiting at lights or junctions, put the car into neutral with the handbrake on. Rest your feet on the floor. It only takes a second to get back into gear again, and you will be less tense when you do so. Occasionally give a slow, gentle push on the steering wheel, using the wrists rather than the whole hand, so that your upper back between the shoulder blades improves its contact with the back of the seat. Pay attention to your elbows. Are they rigid and up in the air? Allow them to be soft and resting easily at your side, pointing down to the floor. Are you gripping the steering wheel too tightly? Relax the fingers and soften the wrists onto the wheel. Imagine you have a glass roof or no roof above your head so you can think about your head going up to the sky. Think about your weight going down into the seat so you are

Staying released while driving improves your speed of reaction.

not holding yourself up off the seat. Are your eyes tense? Is your vision fixed on the car in front? Release the eyes by thinking of what you see coming toward you rather than you going toward it. Remember that you have to consider other road users; otherwise, they will have an accident. Does it matter if you let someone in front of you? Does being another 8 feet/3 meters from the front of the line make any difference? How would you wish to be treated by other road users? Treat other drivers accordingly. Don't get caught up in the tension of being late or in a rush. You can't go any faster than the traffic allows, so think about the present moment and how you are driving rather than your destination and how late you are! If you are already late, another minute makes no difference. Allow yourself to enjoy the drive. Pay attention to your surroundings outside the car.

After the Drive

Sit for a moment before getting out of the car. Swing around gently in your seat and place both feet on the ground before standing slowly by leading with the head. Stand still and allow your feet to release toward the ground while the head goes up to the sky.

Do not peer into the wing mirrors, but let your head rotate to see.

This angle encourages a better use of the lower back and improves the angle between the legs and upper body. The wedge also provides a firm surface to sit on, which gives a better contact through the sitting bones, the two small bones at the base of the pelvis. Many car seats, particularly older ones – are too soft. Older or second hand seats are usually collapsed, very often to one side in particular, through lots of use.

Do not grip the steering wheel.

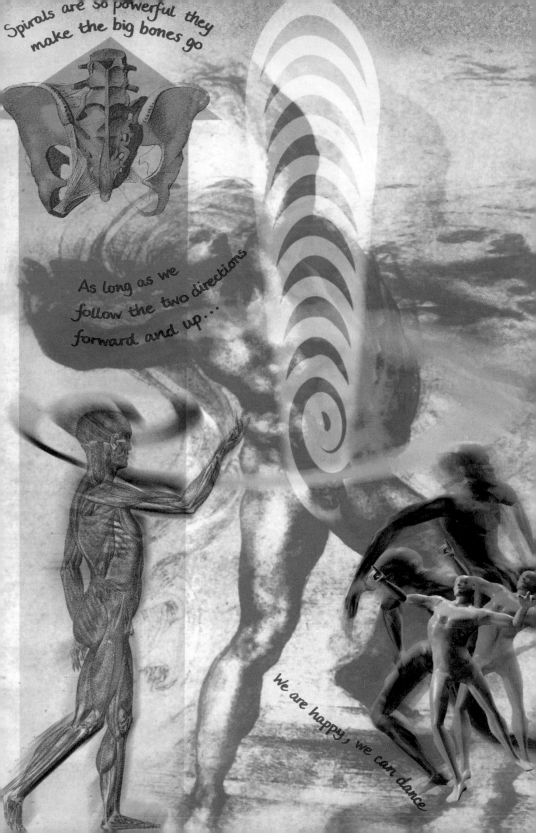

Spirals are so powerful they make the big bones go

As long as we follow the two directions forward and up...

We are happy, we can dance

So we have to wait and think
not to tighten the spirals then
the bones and muscles begin
to want to work again.

PART FOUR

The Universal
Constant in Living

ALEXANDER TECHNIQUE
AND MEDICINE

KNOW THYSELF

BECOME YOURSELF

We have to LET GO
to GET GOING

So we can move again

Spiralling like ever

y else.

Sometimes we can't
dance, so...

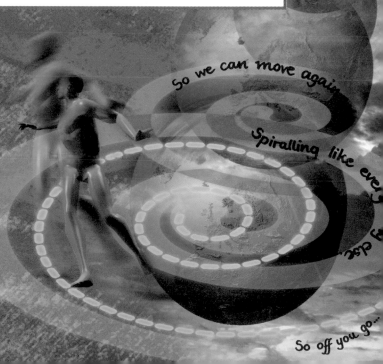

So off you go...

THE UNIVERSAL CONSTANT IN LIVING
ALEXANDER TECHNIQUE AND MEDICINE

Concern is with the sick and convalescent, the aged and crippled. What can be done to prevent the development of physical incapacity and prolong fitness?

INSTITUTE FOR THE ACHIEVEMENT OF HUMAN POTENTIAL

You know that medicines, when well used, restore health to the sick: they will be well used when the doctor, together with his understanding of their nature, shall understand also what man is, what life is, and what constitution and health are.

LEONARDO DA VINCI, *NOTEBOOKS*

THE TECHNIQUE IS PRIMARILY educational in nature, but learning and applying it has therapeutic benefits and preventive consequences for the health of the individual. Alexander was certain that the fact that the dynamic relationship of the head and neck facilitates movement of the whole body could be helpful in diagnosing and treating problems. Many doctors who had lessons with him concurred. In 1937, nineteen doctors urged in the *British Medical Journal* that the Technique be included in medical training.

"We are convinced that Alexander is justified in contending that an unsatisfactory manner of use, by interfering with general functioning, constitutes a predisposing cause of disorder and disease, and that diagnosis of a patient's troubles must remain incomplete unless the medical man when making the diagnosis takes into consideration the influence of use upon functioning. We deplore the fact that this new field of knowledge and experience which has been opened up through Alexander's work has not been investigated by those responsible for the selection of subjects to be studied by medical students."

One of the doctors had said earlier that he believed that the Alexander Technique was not another rival to medicine, but an integral and hitherto overlooked factor.

Doctors are skilled in diagnosing disease and prescribing appropriate drugs or recommending surgical procedures to overcome the pain suffered by their patients. Over the last century, they have begun to study the connection between the functioning of the mind and the body. Psychosomatic illness is recognized by the medical profession as illness induced by the imagination but having no obvious physical symptoms that respond to testing. The importance for medical science of open-minded observation, of "watching and wondering," is becoming popular again.

The Alexander teacher can help you become more aware of your body and how it functions.

Psychosomatic Illness

The word psychosomatic has taken on two meanings in modern speech. On one hand, it refers to something phantom, imagined, perhaps made up, and therefore unreal. In its second sense, it refers to any somatic disorder that is assumed to have at least a partial cognitive or emotional cause. For instance, highly anxious people show a higher incidence of respiratory disorders such as asthma. People in high-pressure, stressful situations show a higher rate of hypertension and gastric dysfunctions. In this sense, the term recognizes that there is a relationship between psychological experience and physiological functioning, that the mind and body interact and have an impact on each other. It appreciates that an illness is no less real because it has a psychological cause. At its most extreme, this position argues that all somatic disorders are, to some degree, rooted in psychological factors.

Alexander teachers are skilled in diagnosing patterns of psychophysical misuse both in themselves and in their students that may limit healthy functioning. They do not diagnose disease, but are looking at dis-ease, the lack of ease that so often leads to malfunctioning. Learning and practicing the Technique is an exploration of how thought affects muscle activity and how muscle activity affects thought.

In particular, patients with the following conditions will benefit from applying the Technique to the extent that the way they use themselves [their cerebral and neuro-muscular systems] is a factor in the genesis and/or continuance of the particular disorder.

In nature, there's no blemish
  but the mind.
None can be called deform'd
  but the unkind.

  WILLIAM SHAKESPEARE: *TWELFTH NIGHT*

- Backache, neckache, where posture is a factor
- Vocal disorders and vocal cord nodules
- Stress
- High blood pressure
- Asthma
- Hyperventilation
- Anxiety states (including performance anxiety)
- Functional disorders
- Osteoarthritis
- Temporo mandibular joint syndrome
- Scoliosis
- Spondylosis
- Migraine
- Tension headaches
- Multiple sclerosis
- Parkinson's disease
- Rehabilitation after stroke, injury, operation, or other treatment
- Dystonias
- Nonspecific regional pain syndrome
- Cerebral palsy

RESETTING THE HOMOEOSTATIC CLOCK

You have inside you a homoeostatic clock, whose job is to maintain the normal/natural state of balance in the body – the status quo. All the actions of the homoeostatic clock are directed toward a state of affairs where there is no need for any further action. It balances and controls the environment of the body.

A very clear example of the operation of the homoeostatic clock is in the ability of the body to maintain a constant temperature. This is a very important part of our healthy survival. Illness is often indicated by "having a temperature," and even an increase of one or two degrees around 98.6°F (37°C) is a sign of an illness and needs to be taken seriously. The opposite is also dangerous, in that if body temperature falls, the condition called hypothermia can

develop. This affects cellular activity, and normal body functioning is impaired, often proving fatal for the very young and the elderly. Most of the heat required to maintain constant body temperature is produced by contraction of muscle fibers. Most of the energy is used up in this reaction, but the energy lost as heat helps maintain the constant level of body temperature. On a very simple level, your hands and feet stay warm – a very beneficial side effect of resetting your homoeostatic clock. When you work with the Alexander Technique, you bring about certain changes in your body structure. This change also affects your homoeostatic clock. The analogy of resetting a clock is an appropriate analogy with what happens as you begin to change and reset yourself through the Alexander Technique procedures.

This change takes place in all the cells of your body. Your muscles, bones, soft tissues – all growing parts of you – accommodate these changes. Your posture and shape change through your new way of thinking.

Every second counts.

CASE STUDY

PROFESSOR NIKOLAAS TINBERGEN
Nobel Prize winner for
Physiology and Medicine,
1973

The claims made by Alexander sounded so extraordinary that I felt I ought to give the method at least the benefit of the doubt. And so, arguing that medical practice often goes by the sound empirical principle of "the proof of the pudding is in the eating," my wife, one of our daughters, and I decided to use the opportunity for observing the effects as critically as we could. For obvious reasons, each of us went to a different Alexander teacher. We discovered that the technique is based on exceptionally sophisticated observation, not only by means of vision but also to a surprising extent by using the sense of touch. It consists in essence of no more than a gentle, at first exploratory, and then corrective manipulation of the entire muscular system. This starts with head and neck, then very soon the shoulders and the chest are involved, and finally the pelvis, legs, and feet, until the whole body is under scrutiny and treatment. As in our own observations of children, the therapist is continually

DEPTH OF SLEEP

monitoring the body and adjusting the procedure all the time. What is actually done varies from one patient to another, depending on what kind of misuse the diagnostic exploration reveals. And naturally, it affects different people in different ways. But between the three of us, we already notice, with growing amazement, very striking improvements in such diverse things as high blood pressure, breathing, depth of sleep, overall cheerfulness, and mental alertness, resilience against outside pressures, and also in such a refined skill as playing a musical instrument. So from personal experience we can already confirm some of the seemingly fantastic claims made by Alexander and his followers, namely that many types of under performance and even ailments, both mental and physical, can be alleviated, sometimes to a surprising extent, by teaching the body musculature to function differently. Although no one would claim that the Alexander treatment is a cure-all in every case, there can be no doubt that it often does have profound and beneficial effects; and, I repeat once more, both in the mental and somatic sphere.

Overall cheerfulness and mental alertness improves.

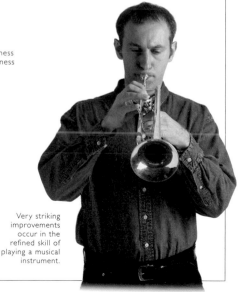

Very striking improvements occur in the refined skill of playing a musical instrument.

BOBATH CLINIC
KATARINA DISS

The following case study is a story of extraordinary dedication and great success. It demonstrates what I have long believed: the Alexander Technique has got something valuable to offer to the cerebral palsy patient who is willing to try this avenue.

Cerebral palsy is a disorder of movement and posture due to a defect or lesion of the immature brain (Brax 1964), whereby the motor development of the cerebral palsy patient is interfered with. Whereas in normal child development we progress quite easily from the fairly gross and uncoordinated movements of a newborn baby to the relatively fine coordination of sitting, crawling, standing, walking as well as eating, talking, and the whole range of manual skills within the first few years of our lives, in the child suffering from cerebral palsy this process is interfered with, bringing about abnormal responses to certain stimuli as well as movements inappropriate to the task intended. These problems can range from being wheelchair bound with severe inability to coordinate the movements of trunk, extremities, head, eye, and mouth to "minor" problems like walking on tiptoes or inability to hold a pencil.

When presented with a stimulus, the cerebral palsy patient has very little, if any, choice to respond in any other but the abnormal (pathological) way. Most forms of physiotherapy dealing with cerebral palsy aim to remedy the situation by trying to teach the patient a different and more varied way of moving.

The Alexander teacher uses his hands as well as words to help his pupil affected by cerebral palsy to become increasingly aware of the moment in time at which the abnormal movement sets in and how to say "No" to it (inhibit the abnormal response). The teacher aims to show the pupil how to achieve a more normal quality of movement by constructively directing his thoughts.

All this will be a gradual process requiring gentle perseverance over several months/years and no miracle cure. Sometimes it may uncover an associated difficulty unrecognized before.

However, as Tony's case study illustrates, it can help to relieve excess tension as well as gradually increase a sense of well-being and ease. There is a good chance of learning something believed impossible before, but above all, it gives the pupil a greater choice by enabling him to say "No" to the unwanted movement.

Balance is interfered with in cerebral palsy.

The crawling stage of development is missed out in many cases of cerebral palsy.

Sitting often presents difficulties for the child with cerebral palsy.

Tony Loyd, an extraordinary success story.

CASE STUDY

Tony Loyd
Computer Consultant

During my birth, I suffered damage to the part of the brain that controlled movement, which resulted in my cerebral palsy. Up to the age of 17 when I left school, I had physiotherapy to help me walk and use my hands, and I had speech therapy. I suffered from the effects of excessive muscular tension. It was hard for me to speak for any length of time, and hard for others to listen to me. Writing and typing for long periods caused back pain. A day's work was tiring.

I had my first lessons in the Alexander Technique nine years ago when I was 25. These weekly lessons, which I have continued with since, showed me what I might be able to achieve. By learning how to focus my attention on breathing out, my breathing became deeper, which made it easier for me to talk, and easier for others to understand me. The lessons made me conscious of a freedom and lightness of movement that I had not had before. I also had the means, by spending time every day lying down, to recreate this sensation and increase my own awareness of it. Whereas before, my life seemed like a mighty climb up a steep and rugged mountain, I could now see life having the ease of a free-flowing run through the long grass on a warm sunny day.

My facility of speech gave me greater self-confidence. The roles I could perform increased, and I was able to pursue a wider range of interests. About 1½ years after having lessons, I was enjoying leading the work of eight people and successfully negotiating the demands of others.

I learned, through the speaking of poetry, how I could use words to express a wide range of feeling. My voice became exciting to use rather than making me frustrated. My finest achievement after attending classes in poetry and public speaking was to perform a two-page stand-up comic routine in an acting class. The success of it, from the laughter it produced and the warm response to it, came from clarity and energy in the voice and stillness in the body.

Difficulties came from releasing the excessive muscular tension. It was like letting go of a taut spring. Occasionally during a lesson or afterward, I had spasms in my right shoulder, which took time to learn how to control. Because this muscular tension had a lot of frustration associated with it, the physical release produced feelings of tearfulness. However, the thought of achieving that freedom and lightness made me determined to overcome these hurdles.

My continued interest in the Technique comes from wanting to take good care of and improve my physical and mental well-being, and to deepen my understanding of how the mind and body interact.

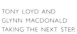

LORD RITCHIE SAID IN THE BRITISH HOUSE OF LORDS ON MAY 9, 1990:

The Technique has been found to be beneficial in numerous ways. It facilitates correct breathing, an essential to health, and eases back problems and refers to the economic as well as the human cost of back pain. It is also thought to be helpful in blood pressure problems, insomnia, and circulation defects. It leads to an upright and most graceful carriage, which is why it is of interest to actors and why most drama schools have the use of an Alexander Technique teacher.

TONY LOYD AND
GLYNN MACDONALD
TAKING THE NEXT STEP.

MEDICAL REFERRALS

Physicians who are well informed about the Technique are happy to refer their patients to Alexander Technique teachers, and such referrals are on the increase as physicians gain more experience of how cost-effective a course of lessons can be in the management of many disorders.

Lessons are available privately or, in the U.K., can be paid for through the National Health Service either in general practice or in some hospitals like St. Bartholomew's or Westmorland. Health insurance in the United States does not usually cover Alexander Technique, though educated physicians do refer patients for lessons. Managed health-care companies in the United States are beginning to recognize the value of non-medical approaches to health. Recognition and acceptance are rapidly growing, and the Alexander Technique is available in many institutions, fitness centers, and wellness centers.

PHYSIOTHERAPISTS FIND THE TECHNIQUE HELPFUL.

A letter in the *British Medical Journal* said:

As practitioners of medicine, we know how great is the need for its (Alexander Technique) resources at the present time, when the strain of existence exacts such a toll even on the healthy. We believe, from practical acquaintance of its effects on ourselves and our patients, that it is adequate to meet that need, if only because it teaches that satisfactory use of the self which is the basis of physical and mental happiness.

Dr. Barlow (1954) demonstrated the re-education procedure with a group of 50 students from the Central School of Speech and Drama in London, England, and reported an improvement for all of them. Speaking as a physician, Dr. Barlow said that he had found the Alexander procedures useful "in such varying conditions as peptic ulcer, spastic colon, ulcerative colitis, eczema, and rheumatoid arthritis" as well as "tension headaches, asthma, low back pain, and fibrositis."

People of all ages can be helped by the Alexander Technique.

PAIN CONTROL

Pain is mysterious and elusive. In *Hard Times* by Charles Dickens, Mrs. Gradgrind gives an answer that strikes a chord with all of us. When asked:

> *"Are you in pain, dear mother?"*
> *"I think there's a pain somewhere in the room,"*
> *said Mrs. Gradgrind, "but I couldn't positively say*
> *that I have got it."*

Dr. Miriam Wohl believes: "It can be a very small difference in functioning that can take someone back over a pain threshold and leave them free of pain. It can make a big difference, especially in the treatment of sciatica." This applies not only to physical pain but in psychological pain – repressed emotions.

Elizabeth Atkinson, Alexander Technique teacher, believes

> *emotion is a moving of the feelings. The problem is*
> *that people are often reluctant to allow their feelings*
> *to move. They get stuck in repetitive situations,*
> *limiting their range of movement on a feeling level.*
> *We talk a lot about not wanting to limit our range of*
> *movement in a physical sense and forget the*
> *psychological realm. The Alexander Technique*
> *enables you to allow the appropriate movement or*
> *deepening of feelings, and so you can begin to*
> *experience the difference between more superficial*
> *responses, for example, embarrassment, cynicism,*
> *flirtatiousness... and deeper, more core responses*
> *such as terror, hatred, sexual passion, and joy.*

PAIN

POSSIBLE FIBROSIS
(BODY LOSES ELASTICITY)

GUARDING MUSCLE SPASM

MYOSITIS
(MUSCLE INFLAMMATION)

BLOOD FLOW

MUSCLE ATROPHY

LACTIC ACID

DECREASED ACTIVITY LEVEL

PAIN

MUSCLE SPASM

Pain cycle used for symptom description by Judy Stern, physical therapist and Alexander Technique teacher.

CASE STUDY

HELENE CORRIE
Mount Vernon Hospital

I have been teaching the Alexander Technique to cancer patients in the Mount Vernon Hospital, London, for the last five years.

I do not consider myself an expert, but have made some interesting observations about the patients that I have seen.

When people are first given the dreaded diagnosis, they experience shock, panic, anger, denial, and always a sense of bereavement and alienation. In many cases the operations they go through leave them disfigured. This deeply affects their perception of themselves and their relationships to their family and friends. Then there is the radiotherapy and chemotherapy, which can cause tiredness, pain, sickness, and breathing difficulties. Through sheer necessity they find resources in themselves they did not know they had. Most of them have a strong will to beat the illness and begin to understand the negative influence of stress on their health. They feel a desire to change.

They come to me as an Alexander teacher to help them make this desire more of a reality. Their lessons make them feel cared for in a human way, experiencing the "one-to-one" relationship and "hands on" touch. They begin to learn a better use of themselves. As a teacher I must not give them false hope, but by learning to improve their use, they begin to have a chance to take part in their recovery. This gives them real hope. The following practical results have been recorded. The patients develop a new awareness of themselves. They stop associating anxiety and pain with pulling down. Improved breathing helps them control panic attacks, insomnia, and the nausea caused by chemotherapy. By learning to move in a more balanced way, the patients gain mobility and save energy. The patients seem to be better equipped to deal with the future, whatever it holds for them.

CASE STUDY

DR. HAGYARD:
Cancer Study

Dr. Hagyard has undertaken a detailed study to assess the benefits of the Alexander Technique on patients with and without the metastatic spread of breast cancer.

I am a physician working in the Oncology Department (treating cancer) at Mount Vernon Hospital, London, and have been working with Helene Corrie, Alexander therapist at the hospital.

Our patient group comprised ten patients, all of whom had a diagnosis of breast cancer, five of whom had suspected or proven distant spread of the disease, and two non-patient members of staff with benign degenerative spinal problems.

My personal impressions and observations are as follows:

• Patients whose reaction to diagnosis was anger, leading to muscle tension, were helped.

• Patients with lung metastases and breathing problems found benefit in ability to use their chest-cage most efficiently and benefited from being in control of breathing.

• It seems to offer those with poor prognosis the opportunity to build in a coping mechanism where later lung or skeletal problems are likely.

• It is best done before symptoms occur, while they are still fit enough to travel and learn. One patient who perhaps had problems before Alexander would undoubtedly have benefited more had she started lessons earlier.

• It helped patients with metastatic spread to learn to have more control and to use their waning powers with 100 percent efficiency.

The receptionist's comment:

"They go in all hunched and tense, and come out straighter and smiling."

KNOW THYSELF

*The fault, dear Brutus, is not in our stars
But in ourselves.*

WILLIAM SHAKESPEARE: JULIUS CAESAR

The unexamined life is not worth living.

SOCRATES

The Alexander Technique invites you to take responsibility for yourself, your thoughts, your actions, how you are feeling, and to realize that you have the power to help yourself. It invites you to recognize that the state you are in largely determines how you perceive yourself and the world around you and that you have the power to change your state. The Technique encourages you to avoid isolating your posture from your thoughts and feelings, but to learn truly to listen to your body and experience it as an indicator about how you are. Through improving the awareness of the body, the self is more able to know itself.

Alexander used the term sensory appreciation to refer to the feedback that we get from our bodies. He also used it to refer to the interrelationships that take place within ourselves: how our thoughts affect our movements and breathing, how our movements affect our feelings, how our emotions can dominate and affect our posture and our capacity for clear thinking. As our sensory appreciation improves, we can become more conscious of how we respond to the constant stimuli from outside and the impulses from inside the self.

DA VINCI
MUNDI

FEAR

Humans have always feared the unknown and lived in constant expectation of an attack from their natural enemies. Although we have moved into a civilized state, this old fear remains. We have developed our mental ability, often to the detriment of our physical prowess. Alexander believed that these imbalances should be addressed and that mankind could become alert and ready to deal with the unknown through becoming more conscious.

There is nothing to fear but fear itself – a trite sound-bite that is more than just a clever cover-up. It has a deep meaning within the very makeup of our neurology.

Most of us go through life as if we were in a permanent state of fear. If your fight-or-flight reaction causes you to have a rigid retracted neck, then the muscles in the neck cannot operate normally. Ideally, the head–neck–back should be operating in a subtle free relationship, allowing lengthening in stature and widening to produce a posture in which optimum breathing is possible. When this relationship is upset, we become stiff, nervous, and tense.

"It is an interesting psychological fact that there are millions of educated people who have cultivated unwillingly the 'worry habit.' This unnecessary worry habit is directly the outcome of the lack of use of our reasoning faculties…"

Children can be seriously affected and the increase in childhood asthma, hypertension, heart attacks, and suicides gives sad evidence to the fact that the way we deal with stress in the psychophysical mechanism is having unacceptable effects. We long for *mens sana in corpore sano*, "a sound mind in a sound body," a phrase that has been used for centuries as an educational goal.

The Alexander Technique teaches you how to overcome your sense of fear by becoming aware of how a rigid, restricted posture has a negative influence on your thoughts and feelings.

FIGHT OR FLIGHT

The short-term stress response called the fight-or-flight response exists to enable us to cope quickly with situations that are life-threatening. In these situations you need extra energy very quickly. The body deals with this need through biological changes. The pulse, blood pressure, and breathing rate all increase to boost energy. More blood is pumped through the blood vessels supplying the muscles, and the bronchial tubes dilate to allow extra air through with each breath. The palms of the hands and the soles of the feet start to perspire – a moist surface provides a better grip. The pupils of the eyes dilate to let in more light and improve vision. Reaction time speeds up. This response is entirely normal and has probably saved our lives on many occasions. To have this response is normal, but to maintain it for long periods is neurotic and unnecessary. When we are stressed we produce cortisol, a hormone that modifies how sensory information is processed. In addition to this hormone, adrenalin is released. One of the quickest ways to reduce cortisol and adrenalin production is to have

All animals use the fight-or-flight response as a means of survival. Humans tend to overmaintain the state.

a good laugh. The biological changes that laughter produces are virtually the reverse of those that occur during a stress response.

The impact that stress has on you depends to a considerable degree upon the ability you have to control it. The Alexander Technique offers you a greater sense of personal control. Even if it were possible, we would not want to eliminate stress completely, as mild, brief, controllable stress can be stimulating and even enjoyable. A controlled amount of adrenalin can positively enhance performance.

Great changes take place in the chemistry of the animal's body when it is threatened.

MALPOSTURE

The startle pattern may be taken as a paradigm of malposture in general, whether it is associated with aging, disease, or lack of exercise. In malposture, muscles in various combinations and degrees of tension have shortened, displacing the head or holding it in a fixed position. Head displacement would have an adverse effect on the rest of the body, partly because of the added weight and the strain put upon muscles and ligaments, but largely, I believe, because of interference in the righting reflexes by abnormal pressure on the joints of the neck. What is basically an incomplete response to gravity would in time come to feel natural, and the muscles contributing to it would be strengthened by exercise.

Startle Pattern Reflex

In *Freedom to Change*, Frank Pierce Jones describes the startle pattern reflex:

> The pattern of startle is remarkably regular. It begins with an eye blink; the head is then thrust forward; the shoulders are raised and the arms stiffened; abdominal muscles shorten; breathing stops, and the knees are flexed. The pattern permits minor variations, but its primary features are the same. Because the startle response is brief and unexpected, it is difficult to observe and more difficult to control. Its chief interest here lies in the fact that it is the model of other, slower response patterns: fear, anxiety, fatigue, and pain all show

Sometimes we enjoy being frightened.

> postural changes from the norm that are similar to those that are seen in startle. In all of them, there is a shortening of neck muscles, which displaces the head, which is usually followed by some kind of flexion response, so that the body is drawn into a slightly smaller space. As in startle, these postural responses cannot take place without the prior displacement of the head and the shortening of the neck muscles. Since these responses are much slower than the startle response, they can be changed by controlling the first stage in the pattern, the head displacement, through which the rest of the pattern is propagated. Changing a response pattern in this way is quite different from suppressing it or ignoring it as a stimulus that may well call for a response. Changing the response pattern simply means that the response will be rational and appropriate to the situation instead of an irrational stereotype. By reorganizing the field of attention, both phases of the response pattern are taken in at the same time. The goal-directed phase (the learned part of the pattern) is allowed to continue, while the set is controlled by the method which I have described. Awareness of the head–neck–trunk relation serves as a framework for the learned activity. By inhibiting the set or fixation of the head, a better distribution of tonus is obtained in the trunk and limbs, and better coordination and control of the specific activity, whether it is speaking or writing or playing the flute.

Sometimes the startle pattern response is the only available response in an extraordinary situation.

MAKING CHOICES

The body reflects the inner disposition of the mind

ROBERT MACDONALD

The Alexander Technique is about making choices in every aspect of your life, from how you behave to becoming the person you want to be. Alexander realized in the early stages of his experiments that he was unable to avoid his tendency to stiffen his neck and shorten his stature when he went to speak. He spent a long time observing himself in the mirror studying his behavior, and eventually he was able to adopt his full stature. However, when he began to recite again, he returned to his old pattern of stiffening and shortening. Alexander realized that the muscular pattern associated with speaking was deeply ingrained and that his new understanding of how to use his body in a free way was overridden by the old pattern. He was still unsuccessful at maintaining an efficient use of himself in the act of speaking. After all this time, his instincts continued to make the old response feel right and natural. So he was finally forced to adopt the following plan:

Throughout our whole life,
from childhood to old age,
we are always making choices.

1. Inhibit any immediate response to the stimulus to speak the sentence.
2. Project in their sequence the directions for the primary control which I had reasoned out as being best for the purpose of bringing about the new and improved use of myself in speaking.
3. Continue to project these directions until I believed I was sufficiently familiar with them to employ them for the purpose of gaining my end and speaking the sentence.
4. While still continuing to project the directions for the new use I would stop and consciously reconsider my first decision and ask myself, "Shall I after all go on to gain the end I have decided upon and speak the sentence? Or shall I not? Or shall I go on to gain some other end all together?", and then and there make a fresh decision:
5. EITHER
   a) not to gain my original end, in which case I would continue to project the directions for maintaining the new use and not go and speak the sentence; OR
   b) to change my end and do something different, or to go on after all and gain my original end, in which case I would continue to project the directions for maintaining the new use to speak the sentence.

What Alexander Did

1. He inhibited his desire to achieve an end.

2. He directed himself into his full and free stature through patient and persistent preparation.

3. He would stop and again ask himself – Shall I speak the sentence, shall I not, or shall I do something different?

4. And then again make a fresh decision either to not speak, to do something different, or to go ahead and speak while continuing to project the directions.

FREDERICK MATTHIAS ALEXANDER

It was only when the conscious options to do, to not do, or to do something different existed up until the moment of action that Alexander overcame his instinctive misdirection. Many of us may find it difficult to break our habitual responses. When we examine our underlying motivation, we may find that we are being driven by the need to get it right, driven by our end-gaining tendency. Our commands to ourselves, however well-meaning, are immediately translated into the need to get it right. As long as we are fixed on getting things right, and getting it right now, we make it impossible for our organism, ourselves, to respond in a new way. We render ourselves inflexible. Our return to our habitual way of performing reflects our mental inflexibility. We assume that our bodies are the problem, but this is not the case. It is the mind that is in a muddle. We can only have choice when there are real alternatives to choose between. Once we have identified clear options in our mind, then the possibility of a new and different response becomes possible. We need to pay attention to the critical moment and practice working with it by becoming more conscious.

When we examine Alexander's method, we may realize that the three options that he put before himself opened up an extremely wide and open landscape for a new response and in so doing had a deep insight into what it means to have "free will."

The Readiness is All

The Alexander Technique helps you to build up the awareness that will help you to apply this strategy to your life. Think of any activity that is important to you, one in which you desire to be at your best and able to respond in the moment to the circumstances as they present themselves. Can you examine your situation in such a way that makes the three options relevant? Think about the alertness of mind that will be required in order to direct the use of yourselves and prepare in the way that Alexander did. Think of the detachment that will be required in order for you to be able to say "No" to your immediate response to the stimulus, and the alertness of mind that will be required to sustain that detachment throughout the situation. And think about the readiness of mind that will be required to make choices in the moment, and even to discover and be open to ones that you have not yet considered.

What do you think this sign says? The literal translation from Chinese is "This Way."

BECOME YOURSELF

Work done with anxiety about results is far inferior to work done without such anxiety, in the calm of self-surrender.
BHAGAVAD GITA

The Alexander Technique began with a man who, through solving his own problems, became able to help others realize that breath is life and life is breath. The Greek word pneuma can mean either breath or spirit. In the Bible, God made man of the dust of the ground, then breathed into his nostrils the breath of life, and he became a living soul. If you stop your breath, you will lose your life. The word "Nirvana" means to breathe out and let go the cares of the world - to stop being anxious, to give a great sigh of relief. We have a chance to make life easier for ourselves, not by dropping out or working harder but by becoming more aware and conscious. Being able to breathe fully allows you to be truly inspired. The word inspiration has two meanings. Physiologically it is breathing in; creatively it is receiving help from the muse. Often we are trapped into a certain way of being because we hold our breath. This can have a damaging effect on our emotional state.

To Thine Own Self Be True

This process works wonderfully when you are unhappy, but it can be used through the day to monitor your state. It gathers you together and helps you in the direction that you choose to go. This way of achieving conscious control over yourself is the great gift of the Alexander Technique. It is not something that you can acquire immediately, for, like all skills, it takes time and practice. You cannot expect to master it immediately, and you need to allow yourself to make mistakes. By beginning to appreciate what is possible and dedicating yourself to the search for personal growth and development, you will unlock the blessing of your conscious mind.

Strategy for Change

1. Stop. Give yourself time and practice conscious inhibition.
2. Pay attention to what is happening. Accept how you are feeling. Open your eyes to the situation as it is now and take responsibility for it.
3. Be aware of your head, neck, and back, and your breathing pattern. Notice the relationship between your postural aspect, your emotional responses, and your thought patterns. Let your sensory appreciation inform of the state of your muscles. Are they locked in old patterns associated with past responses?
4. Ask, "Is this the state in which I want to be?"
5. If the answer is "Yes," then that is what you have chosen.
6. If the answer is "No," then you can choose to change by allowing your neck to be free so your head can go forward and your back can lengthen and widen. Breathe out, then allow the air to return fully, quickly, and freely. Notice the change in your state.

By using your conscious mind, you can begin to come into focus.

BEING ALIVE
The Unity of the Mind,
Body, Spirit

When the mind is free, the body is delicate

WILLIAM SHAKESPEARE: *KING LEAR*

The division of the mind and body is absolutely false. If you begin with dividing the mind and body, you start from a wrong premise, and this false beginning will lead you nowhere. The Alexander Technique helps you to become more conscious of the subtle but critical interactions between the mind and body. As your awareness of posture improves, your ability to feel what is happening in your body increases and you can become more sensitive to the disharmony that occurs in your nervous system as a result of internal and external pressure. From this comes the possibility of avoiding and dealing with stress, heightening your resistance to disease, registering a latent disposition before it turns into overt disease and accelerating the healing process when you have become ill.

Let the neck be free,
let the head go
forward and up.

Definition of the Alexander Technique

The Alexander Technique is not...

1. It is not "curative." It is preventive. "Cures" may take place in the process they are not aimed for.
2. It is not a way of achieving "good" posture.
3. It is not a "treatment."
4. It makes no use of suggestion.
5. It does not have adverse side effects.
6. It is not a "relaxation technique."
7. It is not concerned with remote causes, genetic factors, early experiences, or even medical history.

You have the possibility to help yourself.

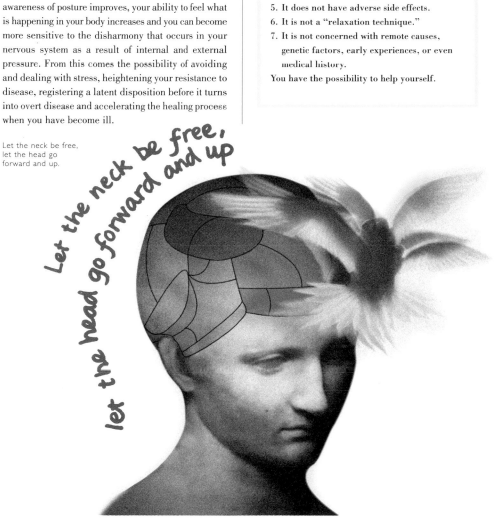

Let the neck be free, let the head go forward and up

TAKING CHARGE OF YOURSELF

Our remedies oft in ourselves do lie
Which we ascribe to heaven; the fated sky
Gives us free scope, only doth backward pull
Our slow designs when we ourselves are dull

WILLIAM SHAKESPEARE, *ALL'S WELL THAT END'S WELL*

Whether we like it or not, the self is always oriented in a particular direction. We may refuse to admit or to pay attention to what our direction is, but we are always in a state of mind and making a decision to remain in that state or to not. Even idleness is a direction - it is the direction of not moving.

Sometimes our direction is positive - we are up, energized, at one with ourselves, making conscious choices and in charge of our direction. At other times we are down, depressed, lacking in optimism, sometimes overwhelmed by negative emotions - bitterness, jealousy, feelings of inadequacy. These feelings often create more conflict because one half of the self wants to be positive, and when we find ourselves responding negatively we get negative about being negative, and the whole situation gets compounded and we find ourselves in a vicious downward spiral. But, nevertheless, we are choosing.

Often these negative cycles are old patterns or habits. One of the definitions of sin is that it is a habit that although once necessary for our survival is no longer so. Perhaps this is the case with some of our negative responses; they are like old skin waiting to be sloughed off. The Alexander Technique is a powerful strategy that can help us deal with the negative actions in our lives.

The light guiding hands of the Alexander Technique teacher help people to find their balance and gain a sense of wholeness.

Achieving your full potential

The Kingdom is inside you, and it is outside you.
When you come to know yourselves, then
you will become known.

GOSPEL OF THOMAS, C.E. 150, FOUND IN 1945 IN EGYPT

There is an old Sufi tale that tells of our search for answers. After the gods had created the world, they decided they would create truth. In order that we humans should not discover it immediately, they had to discover where they should hide truth. Should it be put on the highest mountain, or in the deepest cave, or on the farthest star? All the gods had different ideas as to the best hiding place, but the oldest and wisest god had the best idea. He suggested hiding truth in the very heart of us, knowing that we would look all over the world long before we thought to look inside ourselves.

Getting to know ourselves, coming back in touch, and finding our way are becoming very important to more and more people today. The time has passed when we simply blamed circumstances, birth, or even luck. As we approach the millennium, we are coming to realize that it is we who are the instigators and solvers of our problems. Of course, things happen in our lives that cause us pain and heartache, and we wonder what we have done to be in such a situation. Once we realize that we can help ourselves, often to a surprising degree, we begin to understand and use some proven ways to stop limiting our potential and to begin to gain the ends we want.

The Alexander Technique is a practical way that we can begin this process. For over 100 years, people have been using it as a means whereby to recognize and eventually prevent the habits that hold them back. Through a growing understanding of conscious inhibition and conscious direction, we can learn to give ourselves more time and space in our daily lives. As we grow, we can begin to come into our true inheritance. Hamlet gave us the words; we now have the opportunity to fulfill them.

What a piece of work is a man! How noble in reason!
how infinite in faculty! in form, in moving how
express and admirable! in action how like an angel!
in apprehension how like a god! the beauty of the
world! The paragon of animals.

WILLIAM SHAKESPEARE, *HAMLET*

Autobiography in Five Chapters

I walk down the street
There is a deep hole in the sidewalk
I fall in.
I am lost…I am hopeless.
It isn't my fault.
It takes forever to find a way out.

I walk down the same street.
There is a deep hole in the sidewalk.
I pretend I don't see it.
I fall in again.
I can't believe I am in the same place.
But it isn't my fault.
It still takes a long time to get out.

I walk down the same street.
There is a deep hole in the sidewalk.
I see it is there.
I still fall in…it's a habit.
My eyes are open
I know where I am.
It's my fault.
I get out immediately.

I walk down the same street.
There is a deep hole in the sidewalk.
I walk around it.

I walk down another street.

PORTIA NELSON: *THERE'S A HOLE IN MY SIDEWALK*

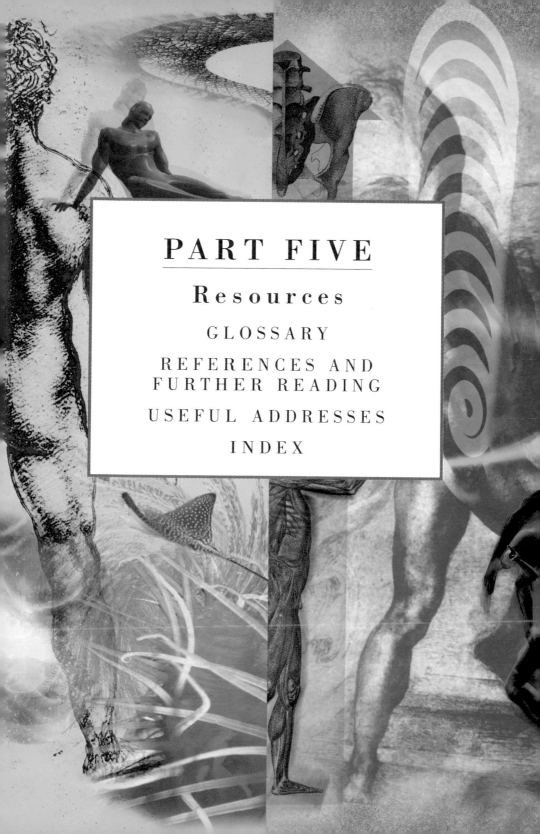

PART FIVE

Resources

GLOSSARY

REFERENCES AND FURTHER READING

USEFUL ADDRESSES

INDEX

GLOSSARY

Abdomen: That portion of the body lying between the thorax and pelvis.

Anatomical position: The body standing erect, face forward, arms at the side and palms forward.

Anoxia: Oxygen deprivation.

Antagonist: A muscle that acts in opposition to another.

Anterior: Toward the front, away from the backbone.

Aphonia: Loss or absence of voice due to failure of vibration of the vocal folds.

Appendicular skeleton: The skeleton of the extremities and of the pectoral and pelvic girdles.

Articulation: Movement and placement of the articulators during speech production.

Axial skeleton: The skeleton of the head and trunk.

Bronchiole: The smallest divisions of the bronchial tree.

Bursa: A sac or saclike cavity.

Cartilage: A nonvascular connective tissue, softer and more flexible than bone.

Chronic: Of long duration.

Clavicle: Collarbone connecting upper extremity to axial skeleton.

Coccyx: The vestigial inferiormost portion of the vertebral column.

Conscious control: The natural faculty that enables us to organize our responses and reflexes in a directed and disciplined way, and so make rational choices in our mental and physical activities.

Cranial: Pertaining to the head.

Diaphragm: The dome-shaped muscle that separates the chest cavity from the abdominal cavity. Attached to the rib cage and flattens out like a trampoline during inspiration, making the area of the lungs bigger.

Directions: The process involved in projecting messages from the brain to the body mechanism to release, lengthen, and widen in conducting the energy necessary to use these mechanisms.

End-gaining: The reaction of trying to achieve an end-result without adequate thought about how the movement is performed, which often leads to unco-ordinated activity.

Eutokia: Happy, relaxed childbirth (classical Greek).

Extension: To increase the angle between bones.

Fiber: A thin strand of nerve or muscle tissue.

Flexion: Decrease the angle between bones.

Harmonic: The partials of a complex sound that are integral multiples of the fundamental frequency.

Inhibition: (1) The learned faculty that allows time to consider how an action is to be performed before proceeding. (2) Essential neurological process.

Inspiration: (1) In physiological terms, the process in which air moves into the lungs. (2) A thought or action that is prompted by divine influence.

Intelligence: The ability to understand and adapt to what is happening in the environment and to be able to use the faculties of learning, memory, and rational choice in making decisions.

Intervertebral: The space between the vertebrae.

Kinesthesia: The sense of movement of muscles, and the perception of weight, resistance, and position.

Ligament: A band of flexible, elastic, dense, fibrous connective tissue connecting the articular ends of bones.

Lumbar: Pertaining to the loin.

Means whereby: The thought given to how an action is achieved. A step-by-step process in which consideration is given to the present conditions, and the need to stop before performing any action. The conscious projection of new directions necessary to the performance of the acts involved in gaining the end.

Neck: (1) The portion of the body that connects the head to the trunk. (2) A narrow portion of any structure serving to join its parts.

Opposition: Moving the thumb to touch the tips of the fingers.

Oxytocin: The hormone released during birth that regulates contractions.

Palate: The roof of the mouth.

Pathology: A biological science dealing with the nature of disease, its courses, and its effects.

Pectoral: Pertaining to the chest.

Pelvis: A basin or basin-shaped cavity.

Perception: The conscious mental registration of a sensory stimulus.

Phalanges: The bones of the fingers and toes.

Physiology: The science of the function of living organisms, or their parts.

Posture: The attitude of the body at any given time. The optimum upright posture is possible if the body is standing at its full height with minimal effort.

Primary control: The balance of the head in relation to the neck and back.

Prone: Lying face down. Opposite of supine.

Proprioceptor: Receptor located in the muscles, tendons, and joints that allows the body to recognize its position.

Psychophysical: The structural and operational relationship of the mind and body.

Reflex: An involuntary, relatively invariable adaptive response to a stimulus.

Resonance: The absorption by a structure of energy at a specific frequency band.

Respiration: The interchange of gases of living matter.

Retract: Draw back, shorten.

Sacrum: The fused vertebrae which, with the coccyx, forms the inferior portion of the vertebral column.

Scapula: The shoulder blade.

Sensation: A change in the state of awareness due to stimulation of an afferent nerve.

Sense organ: A specialized sensory nerve terminal that is activated by a specific stimulus.

Sinus: A cavity or depression within a structure, or existing between two adjacent structures.

Soft palate: The mobile, muscular, posterior portion of the palate that separates the nasal from subjacent cavities.

Somatic: Pertaining to the body and especially the voluntary muscles and skeletal framework.

Spine: Series of vertebrae extending from the skull; the backbone.

Stimulus: Anything that acts as an excitant or irritant for the nervous system.

Supine: Lying on the back, face upward, or the hand with palm upward.

Tendon: A nonelastic band of connective tissue that forms the attachment of muscle to bone.

Thoracic: Pertaining to the thorax.

Thorax: That portion of the torso bounded below by the diaphragm and above by the root of the neck.

Vertebra: One of the bones which forms the vertebral column.

Viscera: The soft internal organs of the body.

Vital capacity: The maximum amount of air that can be exhaled after maximum inhalation.

REFERENCES AND FURTHER READING

Alexander, F.M.
Articles and Lectures Compiled by Jean M.O. Fischer
Mouritz, London, 1995

Alexander, F.M.
Conscious Constructive Control of the Individual
S.T.A.T. Books, London, 1997

Alexander, F.M.
Man's Supreme Inheritance
Mouritz, London, 1996

Alexander, F.M.
The Use of the Self
Gollancz, London, 1996

Alexander, F.M.
The Universal Constant in Living
Chaterson Ltd., 1942

Austin, John H.M., and Ausubel, P.
"Enhanced Respiratory Muskular Functioning in Normal Adults after Lessons in Proprioceptive Muskuloskeletal Education without Exercise" *Chest*, 1992

Barlow, W.
The Alexander Principle
Gollancz, London, 1973

Binkley, G.
The Expanding Self, Edited by Jean M. O. Fischer
S.T.A.T. Books, London, 1993

Brown, R.
Authorized Summaries of F. M. Alexander's Four Books
S.T.A.T. Books, London, 1992

Caplan, D.
Back Trouble
Triad Publishing Co., Gainesville, Florida, 1987

Carrington, W.
A Means of Understanding Man
The Sheildrake Press, London, 1970

Carrington, W.
Thinking Aloud, Edited by Jerry Sontag
Mornum Time Press,
San Francisco, 1994.

Carrington, W., and Carey, S.
Explaining the Alexander Technique: The Writings of F: Matthias Alexander
The Sheildrake Press, London, 1992

Dart, Raymond A.
Skill and Poise
S.T.A.T. Books, London, 1996

De Alcantara, P.
Indirect Procedures: A Musicians' Guide to the Alexander Technique
Oxford University Press,
Oxford, 1997

Jones, F.P.
Freedom to Change: The Development and Science of the Alexander Technique
Mouritz, London, 1997

Garlick, D.
The Lost Sixth Sense, A Medical Scientist Looks at the Alexander Technique
University of New South Wales,
Kensington, 1990

Harris, C.
Fundamentals of Riding: Theory and Practice
Allen and Co., London, 1995

Karlberg, M.
The Neck and Human Balance
Doctoral thesis, Sweden University Hospital, Lund, 1995

Leibowitz, J., Connington, B.
The Alexander Technique
Harper and Row, 1990

Macdonald, G.
Alexander Technique
Hodder and Stoughton,
London, 1994.

Macdonald, R.
The Use of the Voice: Sensory Appreciation, Posture, Vocal Functioning and Shakespearean Text Performance.
Macdonald Media,
London, 1997

Machover, I., Drake, A., & Drake, J.
The Alexander Technique, Birth Book
Sterling Publishing,
New York, London, 1993
Reissued as *Pregnancy and Birth the Alexander Way.*
Robinson Publishing Ltd.,
London, 1995

Maisel, E.
The Resurrection of the Body
Dell Publishing Co., New York, 1969

Roberts, T.D.M.
Understanding Balance: The Mechanics of Posture and Locomotion
Chapman and Hall, London, 1995

Roberts, T.D.M.
"Reflexes, Habits, and Skills"
Paper read at the Constructive Teaching Center, London, 1998

Shaw, S., and D'Angour, A.
The Art of Swimming
Ashgrove Press Limited,
Bath, 1996

Sherrington, C.
The Endeavour of Jean Fernel
Cambridge University Press, Cambridge, 1946

Sherrington, C.
The Integrative Action of the Nervous System
Yale University Press, New Haven, 1961

Tinbergen, N.
"Ethology and Stress Disease" *Science*
Vol 185, 1974

INSTITUTIONS USING THE ALEXANDER TECHNIQUE

London Academy of Music and Dramatic Art

Royal Academy of Dramatic Art

Guildhall School of Music and Drama

Royal National Theatre

Central School of Speech and Drama

Guildford Drama School

Mountview Theatre School

Royal Academy of Music

Royal College of Music

Royal Northern College of Music

Purcell School

Eton College

Westminster Public School

British Association for Performing Arts Medicine

The Menuhin School

Juilliard School

New York University

Metropolitan Opera

Mannes College of Music

The Actor's Studio

The American Academy of Dramatic Arts

Northwestern University School of Music and School of Speech

Indiana University

The Aspen Music Festival and School

New England Conservatory of Music

The Eastman School of Music

USEFUL ADDRESSES

**American Center for the
Alexander Technique (A.C.A.T.)**
129 West 67th Street,
New York City, N.Y. 10023
Tel: 1 212 799 0468

**Alexander Training Institute –
Los Angeles (A.T.I-L.A.)**
1526-14th Street,
Suite 110,
Santa Monica, C.A., 90404
Tel: 1 310 395 9170

**Associaçào Brasileira da
Técnica Alexander (A.B.T.A.)**
Rua dos Miranhas, 333,
Pinheiros, cep: 05434-040,
Sào Paulo - S.P., Brazil

**Assoc. Française des Prof.
Technique Alexander (A.P.T.A.)**
42, Terrasse de l'Iris,
La Défense 2, 92400
Courbevoie, France
Tel: 33 140 90 06 23
Fax: 33 140 90 06 23

**Australian Soc. of Teachers
of the A.T. (A.U.S.T.A.T.)**
PO Box 716,
Darlinghurst,
NSW 2010, Australia
61 08 339 571
(toll free number only within
Australia) 0398 531356

**Belgian Assoc. of Teachers
of F M Alexander Technique
(A.E.F.M.A.T.)**
4 rue des Fonds,
B-1380 Lasne,
Belgium
Tel: 32 2 633 3059

The Brighton Alexander Centre
57 Beaconsfield Villas
Brighton
East Sussex BN1 6HB
Tel: 44 1273 501612
email: nicholls@pavilion.co.uk

**Canadian Society of Teachers
of the A.T. (C.A.N.S.T.A.T.)**
5288 Coolbrook,
Montreal, Quebec H3X 2LI,
Canada
Tel: 1 514 485 6476

**Connington Center for
Performance**
Suite 1i, 123 W. 93rd Street,
New York City, N.Y. 10025
Tel: 1 212 592 1840

**The Constructive
Teaching Centre**
18 Lansdowne Road
London W11
Tel: 44 171 727 7222

**Danish Society of Teachers
of the A.T. (D.F.L.A.T.)**
c/o Michael T. Holm,
Kildebakkegaards Alle 97b,
DK-2860 Soeborg, Denmark
Tel: 45 3969 0330
Fax: 45 86 197434

Eutokia Birth Centre
5 Milman Road
London NW6 6EN
Tel: 44 181 969 5356
email: moshe.machover@kcl.ac.uk

**German Society of Teachers
of the A.T. (G.L.A.T.)**
Postfach 5312,
79020 Freiburg, Germany
Tel: 49 761 383357

**Israeli Society of Teachers
of the A.T. (I.S.T.A.T.)**
PO Box 715,
Karkur 37106, Israel
Tel: 972 6 378244
Fax: 972 6 272211

The Juilliard School
60 Lincoln Center Plaza,
New York City, N.Y. 10023
Tel: 1 212 799 5000

**The London Academy of
Music and Dramatic Art**
266 Cromwell Road
London SW5 0SR
Tel: 44 171 373 9883
email: enquiries@lamda.org.uk
www.lamda.org.uk

Macdonald Media Ltd.
email:
enquiries@macdonaldmedia.co.uk
www.macdonaldmedia.co.uk

Malcolm Balk Running Training
266 Villeneuve West
Montreal, H2V 2RI
Tel: 1 514 843 8032
email: balkm@videotron.com

**Netherlands Society of
Teachers of the A.T.**
Postbus 15591,
1001 NB Amsterdam,
The Netherlands
Tel: 31 20 625 3163

**North American Society of
Teachers of the A.T.
(N.A.S.T.A.T.)**
3010 Hennepin Ave. South,
Suite 10,
Minneapolis, MN 55408,
Tel: 1 612 824 5066

The Royal Academy of Music
Marylebone Road
London NW1 5HT
Tel: 44 171 873 7373
www.ram.ac.uk.

Schiff Action Center
252 West 102nd Street, 1
New York City, N.Y. 10025
Tel: 1 212 222 0176
email: Schiffel@AOL.com

**Society of Teachers of the
Alexander Technique (S.T.A.T.)**
20 London House
266 Fulham Road
London SW10 9EL
Tel: 44 171 351 0828
email: info@stat.org.uk
Statbooks
Tel: 44 171 352 0666
email: statbooks@stat.org.uk

**South African Society of
Teachers of the A.T.
(S.A.S.T.A.T.)**
5 Leinster Road,
Green Point 8001, South Africa
Tel: 27 21 439 3440
Fax: 27 21 439 3440

**Swiss Society of Teachers
of the A.T. (S.V.L.A.T.)**
Postfach, CH-8032 Zürich,
Switzerland
Tel: 41 1 201 03 43

INDEX